Virtual Medical Office

for

Bonewit-West, Hunt, Applegate:
Today's Medical Assistant:
Clinical and Administrative Procedures

Virtual Medical Office

for

Bonewit-West, Hunt, Applegate:
Today's Medical Assistant:
Clinical and Administrative Procedures

Study Guide reviewed by

Susanna M. Hancock, AAS, RMA, CMA, RPT, COLT
AMT Board of Directors
ABHES/ACICS Evaluator
EAI Consultant
Wilder, Idaho

software developed by

Wolfsong Informatics, LLC
Tucson, Arizona

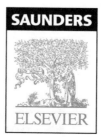

SAUNDERS

ELSEVIER

SAUNDERS
ELSEVIER

11830 Westline Industrial Dr.
St. Louis, Missouri 63146

VIRTUAL MEDICAL OFFICE FOR
BONEWIT-WEST, HUNT, APPLEGATE:
TODAY'S MEDICAL ASSISTANT: CLINICAL AND ADMINISTRATIVE PROCEDURES
FIRST EDITION

ISBN: 978-1-4160-5265-4

Copyright © 2009 by Saunders, an imprint of Elsevier Inc.

Some material was previously published.

Although for mechanical reasons all pages of this publication are perforated, only those pages
imprinted with an Elsevier Inc. copyright notice are intended for removal.

Notice

Knowledge and best practice in this field are constantly changing. As new research and experience
broaden our knowledge, changes in practice, treatment and drug therapy may become necessary or
appropriate. Readers are advised to check the most current information provided (i) on procedures
featured or (ii) by the manufacturer of each product to be administered, to verify the recommended
dose or formula, the method and duration of administration, and contraindications. It is the
responsibility of the practitioner, relying on their own experience and knowledge of the patient, to
make diagnoses, to determine dosages and the best treatment for each individual patient, and to
take all appropriate safety precautions. To the fullest extent of the law, neither the Publisher nor
the Authors assumes any liability for any injury and/or damage to persons or property arising out
or related to any use of the material contained in this book.

ISBN: 978-1-4160-5265-4

Acquisitions Editor: Susan Cole
Managing Editor: Scott Weaver
Senior Developmental Editor: Donna Morrissey
Publishing Services Manager: Linda McKinley
Senior Project Manager: Stephen Bancroft
Cover Designer: James Almond

Printed in the United States of America

Last digit is the print number: 9 8 7 6 5 4 3

Table of Contents

Getting Started

GETTING SET UP

■ **RECOMMENDED SYSTEM REQUIREMENTS**

WINDOWS®

Windows PC
Windows XP, Windows Vista™
Pentium® processor (or equivalent) @ 1 GHz (Recommend 2 GHz or better)
1.5 GB hard disk space
512 MB of RAM (Recommend 1 GB or more)
CD-ROM drive
800 x 600 screen size
Thousands of colors
Soundblaster 16 soundcard compatibility
Stereo speakers or headphones

MACINTOSH®

Virtual Medical Office is not compatible with the Macintosh platform.

■ **INSTALLATION INSTRUCTIONS**

WINDOWS

1. Insert the *Virtual Medical Office* CD-ROM.
2. Inserting the CD should automatically bring up the setup screen if the current product is not already installed.
   a. If the setup screen does not appear automatically (and *Virtual Medical Office* has not been installed already), navigate to the "My Computer" icon on your desktop or in your Start menu.
   b. Double-click on your CD-ROM drive.
   c. If installation does not start at this point:
      (1) Click the **Start** icon on the task bar and select the **Run** option.
      (2) Type d:\setup.exe (where "d:\" is your CD-ROM drive) and press **OK**.
      (3) Follow the onscreen instructions for installation.
3. Follow the onscreen instructions during the setup process.

1

■ HOW TO LAUNCH VIRTUAL MEDICAL OFFICE

WINDOWS

1. Double-click on the *Virtual Medical Office* icon located on your desktop.
2. Or navigate to the program via the Windows Start menu.

■ SCREEN SETTINGS

For best results, your computer monitor resolution should be set at a minimum of 800 x 600. The number of colors displayed should be set to "thousands or higher" (High Color or 16 bit) or "millions of colors" (True Color or 24 bit).

WINDOWS

1. From the **Start** menu, select **Settings**, then **Control Panel**.
2. Double-click on the **Display** icon.
3. Click on the **Settings** tab.
4. Under **Screen resolution** use the slider bar to select **800 by 600 pixels**.
5. Access the **Colors** drop-down menu by clicking on the down arrow.
6. Select **High Color (16 bit)** or **True Color (24 bit)**.
7. Click on **OK**.
8. You may be asked to verify the setting changes. Click **Yes**.
9. You may be asked to restart your computer to accept the changes. Click **Yes**.

■ TECHNICAL SUPPORT

Technical support for this product is available between 7:30 a.m. and 7 p.m. (CST), Monday through Friday. Before calling, be sure that your computer meets the system requirements to run this software. Inside the United States and Canada, call 1-800-692-9010. Outside North America, call 314-872-8370. You may also fax your questions to 314-523-4932 or contact Technical Support through e-mail: technical.support@elsevier.com.

Trademarks: Windows, Pentium, and America Online are registered trademarks.

ACCESSING *Virtual Medical Office Online Study Guide*
ON EVOLVE

The product you have purchased is part of the Evolve family of online courses and learning resources. Please read the following information thoroughly to get started.

To access the *Virtual Medical Office Online Study Guide* on Evolve:

Your instructor will provide you with the username and password needed to access the *Virtual Medical Office Online Study Guide* on the Evolve Learning System. Once you have received this information, please follow these instructions:

1. Go to the Evolve login page (http://evolve.elsevier.com/login).

2. Enter your username and password in the **Login to My Evolve** area and click the arrow or hit **Enter**.

3. You will be taken to your personalized **My Evolve** page, where the course will be listed in the **My Courses** module.

TECHNICAL REQUIREMENTS

To use the *Virtual Medical Office Online Study Guide*, you will need access to a computer that is connected to the Internet and equipped with web browser software that supports frames. For optimal performance, it is recommended that you have speakers and use a high-speed Internet connection. However, slower dial-up modems (56 K minimum) are acceptable.

■ WEB BROWSERS

Supported web browsers include Microsoft Internet Explorer (IE) version 6.0 or higher and Mozilla Firefox version 2.0 or higher.

If you use America Online® (AOL) for web access, you will need AOL version 4.0 or higher and one of the browsers listed above. Do not use earlier versions of AOL with earlier versions of IE, because you will have difficulty accessing many features.

For best results with AOL:
- Connect to the Internet using AOL version 4.0 or higher.
- Open a private chat within AOL (this allows the AOL client to remain open, without asking whether you wish to disconnect while minimized).
- Minimize AOL.
- Launch a recommended browser.

Whichever browser you use, the browser preferences must be set to enable cookies and JavaScript and the cache must be set to reload every time.

Enable Cookies

Browser	Steps
Internet Explorer (IE) 6.0 or higher	1. Select **Tools → Internet Options**. 2. Select **Privacy** tab. 3. Use the slider (slide down) to **Accept All Cookies**. 4. Click **OK**. -OR- 3. Click the **Advanced** button. 4. Click the check box next to **Override Automatic Cookie Handling**. 5. Click the **Accept** radio buttons under **First-party Cookies** and **Third-party Cookies**. 6. Click **OK**.
Mozilla Firefox 2.0 or higher	1. Select **Tools → Options**. 2. Select the **Privacy** icon. 3. Click to expand Cookies. 4. Select **Allow sites to set cookies**. 5. Click **OK**.

Enable JavaScript

Browser	Steps
Internet Explorer (IE) 6.0 or higher	1. Select **Tools → Internet Options**. 2. Select **Security** tab. 3. Under **Security level for this zone** set to **Medium** or lower.
Mozilla Firefox 2.0 or higher	1. Select **Tools → Options**. 2. Select the **Content** icon. 3. Select **Enable JavaScript**. 4. Click **OK**.

Set Cache to Always Reload a Page

Browser	Steps
Internet Explorer (IE) 6.0 or higher	1. Select **Tools → Internet Options**. 2. Select **General** tab. 3. Go to the **Temporary Internet Files** and click the **Settings** button. 4. Select the radio button for **Every visit to the page** and click **OK** when complete.
Mozilla Firefox 2.0 or higher	1. Select **Tools → Options**. 2. Select the **Privacy** icon. 3. Click to expand Cache. 4. Set the value to "0" in the **Use up to: __ MB of disk space for the cache** field. 5. Click **OK**.

Plug-Ins

Adobe Acrobat Reader—With the free Acrobat Reader software, you can view and print Adobe PDF files. Many Evolve products offer student and instructor manuals, checklists, and more in this format!

Download at: http://www.adobe.com

Apple QuickTime—Install this to hear word pronunciations, heart and lung sounds, and many other helpful audio clips within Evolve Online Courses!

Download at: http://www.apple.com

Adobe Flash Player—This player will enhance your viewing of many Evolve web pages, as well as educational short-form to long-form animation within the Evolve Learning System!

Download at: http://www.adobe.com

Adobe Shockwave Player—Shockwave is best for viewing the many interactive learning activities within Evolve Online Courses!

Download at: http://www.adobe.com

Microsoft Word Viewer—With this viewer Microsoft Word users can share documents with those who don't have Word, and users without Word can open and view Word documents. Many Evolve products have testbank, student and instructor manuals, and other documents available for downloading and viewing on your own computer!

Download at: http://www.microsoft.com

Microsoft PowerPoint Viewer—View PowerPoint 97, 2000, and 2002 presentations even if you don't have PowerPoint with this viewer. Many Evolve products have slides available for downloading and viewing on your own computer!

Download at: http://www.microsoft.com

SUPPORT INFORMATION

Live support is available to customers in the United States and Canada from 7:30 a.m. to 7 p.m. (CST), Monday through Friday by calling **1-800-401-9962**. You can also send an email to evolve-support@elsevier.com.

There is also **24/7 support information** available on the Evolve website (http://evolve.elsevier.com), including:

- Guided Tours
- Tutorials
- Frequently Asked Questions (FAQs)
- Online Copies of Course User Guides
- And much more!

Office Tour

Welcome to *Virtual Medical Office*, a virtual office setting in which you can work with multiple patient simulations and also learn to access and evaluate the information resources that are essential for providing high-quality medical assistance.

In the virtual medical office, Mountain View Clinic, you can access the Reception area, Exam Room, Laboratory, Office Manager, and Check Out area, plus a separate room for Billing and Coding.

■ BEFORE YOU START

Make sure you have your textbook nearby when you use the *Virtual Medical Office* CD. You will want to consult topic areas in your textbook frequently while working with the CD and using this study guide.

■ HOW TO SIGN IN

- Double-click on the *Virtual Medical Office* icon on your computer's desktop to start the program.
- Once the software has loaded, enter your name on the Medical Assistant identification badge
- Click on **Start Simulation**.

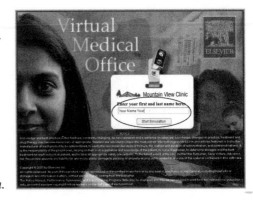

Enter your name and click Start Simulation.

- This takes you to the office map screen. Across the top of this screen is the list of patients available for you to follow throughout their office visit.

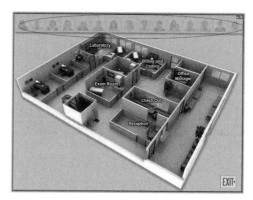

Office map with patient list.

■ PATIENT LIST

1. **Janet Jones (age 50)**—Ms. Jones has sustained an on-the-job injury. She is in pain and impatient. By working with Ms. Jones, students will learn about managing difficult patients, as well as the requirements involved in Workers' Compensation cases.

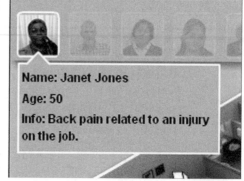

Janet Jones

2. **Wilson Metcalf (age 65)**—A Medicare patient, Mr. Metcalf is being seen for multiple symptoms of abdominal pain, nausea, vomiting, and fever. He is seriously ill and might need more specialized care in a hospital setting.

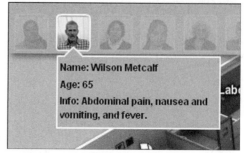

Wilson Metcalf

3. **Rhea Davison (age 53)**—An established patient with chronic and multiple symptoms, Ms. Davison does not have medical insurance.

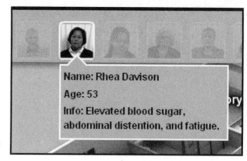

Rhea Davison

4. **Shaunti Begay (age 15)**—A new patient, Shaunti Begay is a minor who has an appointment for a sports physical. Upon arrival, Shaunti and her family learn that Mountain View Clinic does not participate in their health insurance.

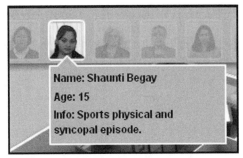

Shaunti Begay

5. **Jean Deere (age 83)**—Accompanied by her son, Ms. Deere is an established Medicare patient being evaluated for memory loss and hearing loss.

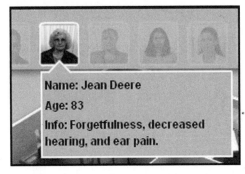

Jean Deere

6. **Renee Anderson (age 43)**—Ms. Anderson scheduled her appointment for a routine gynecologic exam but exhibits symptoms that suggest she is a victim of domestic violence.

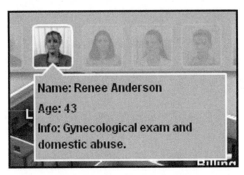

Renee Anderson

7. **Teresa Hernandez (age 16)**—Teresa is a minor patient who is unaccompanied by a parent for her appointment. She is seeking contraceptive counseling and STD testing.

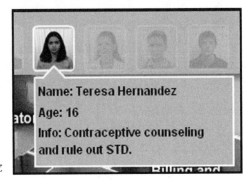

Teresa Hernandez

8. **Louise Parlet (age 24)**—Ms. Parlet is an established patient being seen for a pregnancy test and examination. She will also need to be referred to an OB/GYN specialist.

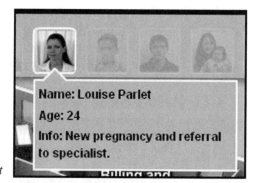

Louise Parlet

9. **Tristan Tsosie (age 8)**—A minor patient accompanied by his older sister and younger brother, Tristan is having a splint and sutures removed from his injured right arm.

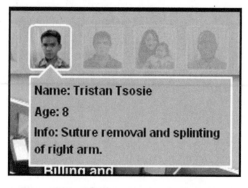

Tristan Tsosie

10. **Jose Imero (age 16)**—Jose is a minor patient who is scheduled for an emergency appointment to have the laceration on his foot sutured.

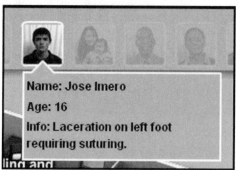

Jose Imero

11. **Jade Wong (age 7 months)**—Jade and her parents are new patients to Mountain View Clinic. Jade needs a checkup and updates to her immunizations. Her mother does not speak English.

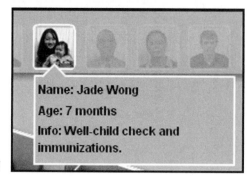

Jade Wong

12. **John R. Simmons (age 43)**—Dr. Simmons is a new patient with a history of high blood pressure and recent episodes of blood in his urine.

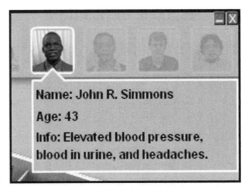

John R. Simmons

13. **Hu Huang (age 67)**—Mr. Huang developed a severe cough and fever after returning from a recent trip to Asia.

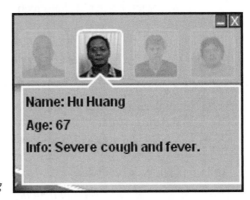

Hu Huang

14. **Kevin McKinzie (age 18)**—Mr. McKinzie has made an appointment because of his nausea and vomiting. He is insured through the restaurant where he works.

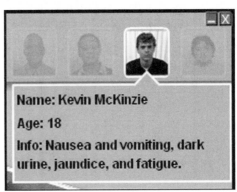

Kevin McKinzie

15. **Jesus Santo (age 32)**—Mr. Santo has been brought to the office as a walk-in appointment by his employer for leg pain and a fever. He has no insurance or identification, but his employer has offered to pay for the visit.

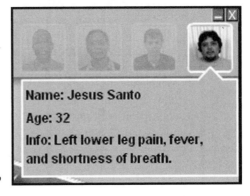

Jesus Santo

◼ BASIC NAVIGATION

HOW TO SELECT A PATIENT

The list of patients is located across the top of the office map screen. Pointing your cursor at the various patients will highlight their photo and reveal their name, age, and medical problem (see examples in the photos on the previous pages). When you click on the patient you wish to review, a larger photo and description will appear in the lower left corner of the screen.

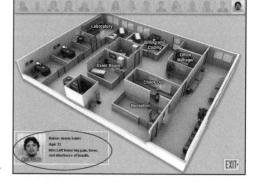

Click on a photo to select a patient.

Note: You **must** select a patient before you are allowed access to the Reception area, Exam Room, Laboratory, Billing and Coding office, or Check Out area. The Office Manager area is the only room you can enter without first selecting a patient.

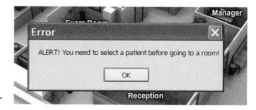

Select a patient before choosing a room.

HOW TO SELECT A ROOM

After selecting a patient, use your cursor to highlight the room you want to enter. The active room will be shaded blue on the map. Click to enter the room.

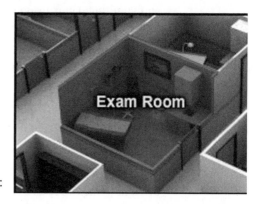

Highlight and click on a room to enter.

HOW TO LEAVE A ROOM

When you are finished working in a room, you can leave by clicking the exit arrow found at the bottom right corner of the screen.

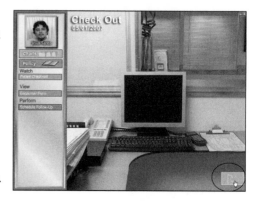

Click on the exit arrow.

Leaving a room will automatically take you to the Summary Menu.

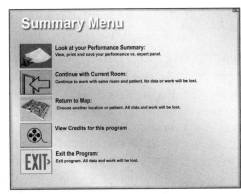

The Summary Menu

From the Summary Menu, you can choose to:

- **Look at Your Performance Summary**

  In each room there are interactive wizards or tasks that can be completed. The Performance Summary lets you compare your answers with those of the experts.

- **Continue with Current Room**

  This takes you back to the last room in which you worked. This option is not available if you have already reviewed your Performance Summary.

- **Return to Map**

  This reopens the office map for you to select another room and/or another patient.

- **View Credits for This Program**

  This provides a complete listing of software developers, publisher, and authors.

- **Exit the Program**

  This closes the *Virtual Medical Office* software. You will need to sign in again before you can use the program.

HOW TO USE THE PERFORMANCE SUMMARY

If you completed any of the interactive wizards in a room, you can compare your answers with those of the experts by accessing your Performance Summary. The Performance Summary is not a grading tool, although it is valuable for self-assessment and review.

From the Summary Menu, click on **Look at Your Performance Summary**.

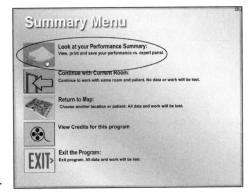

Select Look at Your Performance Summary.

The complete list of tasks associated with the active room will appear with two columns showing the results of your choices. Your answers will appear in the column labeled **Your Performance**, and the answers chosen by the expert will appear in the **Expert's Performance** column. A check mark in the same box in both columns indicates that your answer matched the expert's answer. The Performance Summary can be saved to your computer or disk by clicking on the disk icon at the upper right side of the screen. The saved file can be printed or e-mailed to your instructor. A hard copy can also be printed without saving by clicking on the printer icon at the upper right corner of the screen.

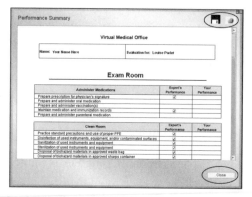

The Performance Summary can be printed and/or saved.

ROOM DESCRIPTIONS

Each room can be entered at any time in any order. You can follow a patient's visit from Reception to Check Out, or you can choose to observe each patient at any point in their care. Below is a description of the information and activities that can be found in various rooms.

ALL ROOMS

- In all rooms you can access the patient's medical record and the office Policy Manual.

- In all rooms in which there are interactive tasks to be completed, you can select tasks or features from the menu on the left of the screen, as shown on this sample of the menu in the Reception area.

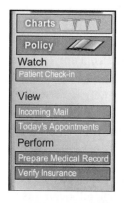

Reception area menu

- As an alternative to using the menu, you can click on the corresponding items in the photo of the room. As you move your cursor over each item connected to one of the tasks on the menu, it will highlight and become active.

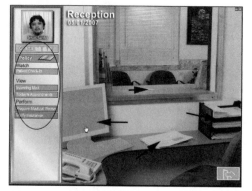

Reception area

RECEPTION

In the Reception area, you can choose:

- **Charts**—Look at the patient's chart. *Note:* For new patients, there will be no information available in the chart at this time although you do have the option of assembling a new medical record.
- **Policy**—Open the office Policy Manual and review the established administrative, clinical, and laboratory policies for Mountain View Clinic. Within the Policy Manual you will also find the Coding and Billing Manual.
- **Watch**—Watch a video of the patient's arrival. Each patient is shown checking in at the front desk so that you can observe the procedures typically performed by the receptionist and consider some of the various problems that might arise.
- **Incoming Mail**—Look at the incoming mail for the day. Mountain View Clinic has received a wide range of correspondence that must be read and responded to accordingly.
- **Today's Appointments**—Review the appointment schedule for the day. You can check the schedule to find out what time patients are supposed to arrive, the reason for their visit, and how much time the physician will need for the examination.
- **Prepare Medical Record**—Practice preparing the medical record. This interactive feature allows you to build a medical record for a new patient or update information for an established patient.
- **Verify Insurance**—Verify a patient's insurance. Also interactive, this feature allows you to ask patients about the status of their insurance and to view their insurance cards.

EXAM ROOM

- **Charts** and **Policy**—Access the patient's chart and the office Policy Manual.
- **Watch**—View video clips of different parts of the patient's exam. Observe the actions of the medical assistants in the videos and critique the competencies demonstrated.
- **Exam Notes**—Review the physician's documented findings for the current visit. These notes are added to the full Progress Notes in the patient's chart as the patient continues on to Check Out.
- **Perform**—Perform multiple tasks that are required of a clinical medical assistant, such as preparing the room for the exam, taking vital signs and patient history, and properly positioning the patient for an exam.

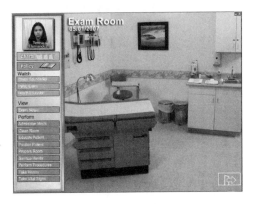

LABORATORY

- **Charts** and **Policy**—Access the patient's chart and the office Policy Manual.
- **View: Logs**—View the laboratory's log of specimens sent out for testing. Opportunities to practice filling out laboratory logs are included in the workbook exercises.
- **Perform**—Perform specific tasks as needed in the laboratory, such as collecting and testing specimens. These interactive wizards walk you through the steps for collecting and testing specimens ordered by the physician as part of the patient's examination. The Progress Notes are available throughout so that you can review the physician's directions.

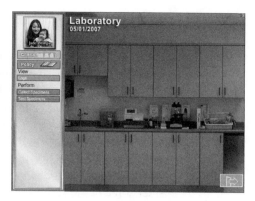

CHECK OUT

- **Charts** and **Policy**—Access the patient's chart and the office Policy Manual.
- **Watch**—Watch a video clip of the patient checking out of the office at the end of the visit. Observe the administrative medical assistants as they schedule follow-up appointments, accept payments, and manage the various duties and problems that may arise.
- **View**—Look at the Encounter Form completed for each patient and verify that the form is filled out correctly and completely.
- **Perform**—Certain patients will require a return visit to the office. Schedule their follow-up appointments as needed. Opportunities to work with the appointment book and additional scheduling tasks are included in the study guide.

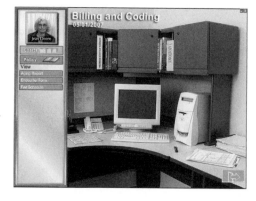

BILLING AND CODING

- **View: Aging Report**—Review the outstanding balances on various patient accounts and assess when to implement different collection techniques.
- **View: Encounter Form**—Review the patient's Encounter Form and determine whether the proper procedures were followed to ensure accurate billing and coding.
- **View: Fee Schedule**—Review the office's fee schedule to calculate the proper charges for the patient's visit.

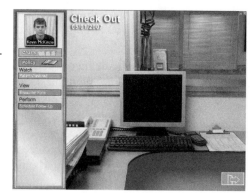

OFFICE MANAGER

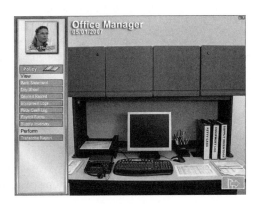

- **Policy**—View the office Policy Manual. Note that patient charts are not available from the manager's office, and there is no need to select a patient to enter the Office Manager area.
- **View**—A variety of financial and administrative documents are available for viewing in the manager's office. Banking deposits and payments can be tracked through these documents, and opportunities to practice managing office finances are included in the study guide.
- **Perform: Transcribe Report**—A recorded medical report is included for transcription practice with full player controls.

■ EMBEDDED ERRORS

The individual lessons and patient scenarios associated with the *Virtual Medical Office* program were designed to stimulate critical thinking and analytical skills and to help develop the competencies you will be tested on as part of your course work. Thus deliberate errors have been embedded into each of the 15 patient scenarios and in the Billing and Coding and Office Manager activities. Many of the exercises in the study guide draw attention to these errors so that you can work through how and why a correction needs to be made. Other errors have not been specifically addressed, and you may discover them as you work through the various rooms and tasks. Instructors and students alike are encouraged to use any errors they find to further develop the essential critical thinking and decision-making skills needed for the clinical office.

The following icons are used throughout the study guide to help you quickly identify particular activities and assignments:

 Reading Assignment—tells you which textbook chapter(s) you should read before starting each lesson

 Writing Activity—certain activities focus on written responses such as filling out forms or completing documentation

 CD-ROM Activity—marks the beginning of an activity that uses the *Virtual Medical Office* simulation software

 CD-ROM Instructions—indicates the steps to follow as you navigate through the software

 Reference—indicates questions and activities that require you to consult your textbook

 Time—indicates the approximate amount of time needed to complete the exercise

LESSON 1

The Health Care System and the Professional Medical Assistant

✐ **Reading Assignment:** Chapter 1—The Health Care System

Chapter 2—The Professional Medical Assistant

Patient: Rhea Davison

Objectives:

- Identify the flow of activity in ambulatory care.
- Identify the various types of health care professionals.
- List and describe the parts of the medical office.

Exercise 1

 CD-ROM Activity—Flow of Activity

 10 minutes

- Sign in to Mountain View Clinic and review the office map.

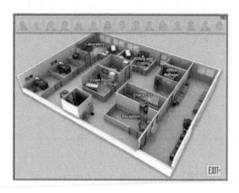

The office map

1. The patient list, which appears above the office map, shows the various patients who will be seen at Mountain View Clinic. Because there are multiple patients coming to the clinic to

   receive treatment, Mountain View Clinic is best described as an _____ care office.

2. Listed below are the various rooms used by Mountain View Clinic. Based on what you read in the textbook chapter, identify the order in which the rooms will be used for patient care.

Room	**Order Used**
_____ Exam Room	a. First
_____ Billing and Coding	b. Second
_____ Reception	c. Third
_____ Office Manager	d. Fourth
_____ Check Out	e. Fifth
_____ Laboratory	f. Sixth

Exercise 2

 CD-ROM Activity—Health Care Professionals

15 minutes

- From the patient list at the top of the office map, select **Rhea Davison**.

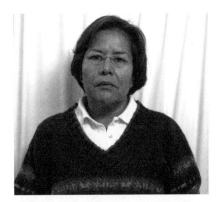

Rhea Davison

- On the office map, highlight and click on **Reception**.

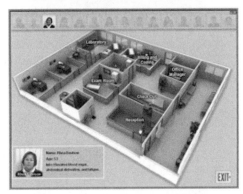

Click on Reception.

- To open the Policy Manual, select **Policy** from the menu on the left side of the screen.

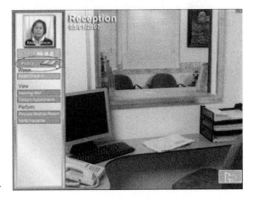

Click on Policy.

- When the Policy Manual opens, type "job descriptions" in the search bar.
- Click the magnifying glass and read through the job descriptions identified for Mountain View Clinic.

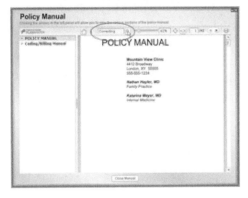

1. Match the specific duties listed below to the appropriate job title of the person who performs those duties. (*Hint:* You may use job titles more than once.)

Duties	Job Title
_____ Prepares patients and rooms to be used for exams, treatments, minor surgeries, and diagnostic tests	a. Office Manager
	b. Clinical Medical Assistant
_____ Assembles all patient records for each day's appointments	c. Administrative Medical Assistant
	d. Biller/Coder
_____ Schedules employees' work	
_____ Monitors compliance with all federal, state, and local statutes	
_____ Performs CLIA-waived diagnostic tests	
_____ Files all insurance claims according to appropriate third-party guidelines	
_____ Transcribes dictated medical documents	
_____ Mails monthly accounts receivable statements	
_____ Obtains managed care precertifications for patient procedures and/or treatments	

→ • Close the Policy Manual to return to the Reception desk.

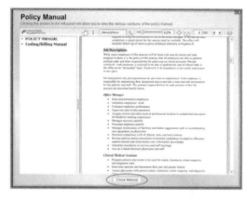

Click Close Manual.

• Remain in the Reception area with Rhea Davison and select **Patient Check-In** to watch the video of Ms. Davison's arrival at Mountain View Clinic.

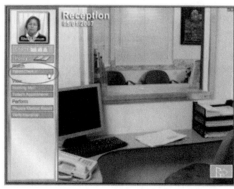

Click on Patient Check-In.

• At the end of the video, click **Close** to return to Reception.

2. In the video, the medical assistant discusses the CMA credential. However, the RMA is another credential that is recognized on a national level. What does RMA stand for, and what is the accrediting agency? (*Hint:* Use the Internet and any other available resources.)

3. On arrival this morning, Dr. Meyer states that you need to check on her medical license renewal, because it has not arrived and her current license expires on June 1. Go to the Internet and find the name and address of the medical examining board for the state in which you live. Also find the time limit for medical licensure and any necessary components for renewal of the license. Print your findings for your instructor.

➤ • Remain in the Reception area with Ms. Davison and continue to the next exercise.

Exercise 3

 CD-ROM Activity—Parts of the Medical Office

 15 minutes

- Remain in the Reception area with Rhea Davison as your patient. (*Note:* If you have exited the program, sign back in to Mountain View Clinic and select Rhea Davison from the patient list.)
- Take a minute to become more familiar with the Reception area by using your mouse to roll over the different items in the room.

1. Which of the following items are necessary to have in a Reception area? Select all that apply.

_____ Weight scale with height bar

_____ Telephone

_____ Hazardous waste container

_____ Appointment book or computer for scheduling

_____ Patient charts

_____ Thermometer

_____ Mail

_____ Chairs

_____ Patient information and HIPAA forms

_____ Blood pressure cuff

2. Earlier, when you watched the video of Ms. Davison's check-in, what information did Kristin, the receptionist, neglect to collect from Ms. Davison?

Ethics and Law for the Medical Office

Reading Assignment: Chapter 3—Ethics and Law for the Medical Office

Patient: Wilson Metcalf

Objectives:

- Recognize a potential liability problem and identify the possible solutions.
- Identify breaches of medical ethics and etiquette at Mountain View Clinic.
- Determine the appropriate actions or behaviors to ensure that medical ethics and etiquette standards are met.

Exercise 1

 CD-ROM Activity—General Liability

 20 minutes

- Sign in to Mountain View Clinic.
- Select **Wilson Metcalf** from the patient list.

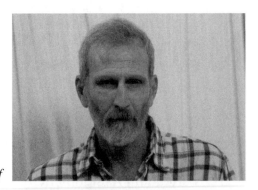

Wilson Metcalf

- On the office map, highlight and click on **Reception**.

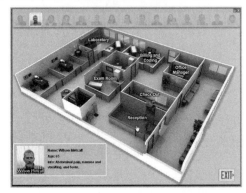

Click on Reception.

- Click on **Policy** to open the office Policy Manual.

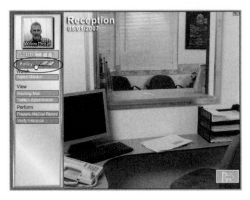

Click on Policy.

- Expand the Policy Manual's table of contents by clicking on the arrow next to **Policy Manual** located on the menu to the left.

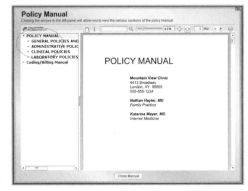

Click arrow to expand.

- Click on **Administrative Policies** and then on **Emergency Office Guidelines**. Read pages 17-19 of the Policy Manual.
- Click on **Close Manual** to return to the Reception Desk.

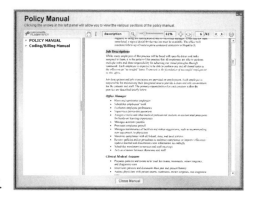

Click on Close Manual.

- Click on **Patient Check-In** (under Watch) to view the video of Mr. Metcalf's arrival at Mountain View Clinic.

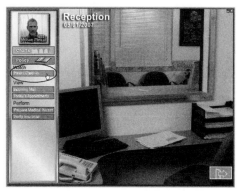

Click on Patient Check-In.

1. As you watched the video, what did you observe about Mr. Metcalf's condition?

2. Based on your observations, was it appropriate for Kristin to keep Mr. Metcalf at the counter while she completed the check-in process? Explain your answer.

3. What was the rationale for Kristin to close the window? Was it appropriate for her to close the window at this time? Why or why not?

4. Did Kristin leave herself and the practice open to any potential liability issue(s) in this scene? If so, describe the issue(s) you identified.

5. Describe any other potential liability issues involving any of the other medical staff appearing in this video.

6. If Mr. Metcalf had been injured as a result of his fall and the subsequent treatment by the office staff and he chose to pursue legal action against the practice, who would be at risk for liability?
   a. The physicians, the practice, and all three medical assistants
   b. The practice, Charlie, and Kristin
   c. Only Charlie and Kristin
   d. Only Kristin

7. What alternative actions could Kristin and the office staff have taken that would have avoided the potential liability issue(s) already identified? List at least five actions.

→ • Click **Close** to return to the Reception desk.

Exercise 2

 CD-ROM Activity—Breaches of Medical Ethics and Medical Etiquette

 10 minutes

- Remain in the Reception area with Wilson Metcalf as your patient. (*Note:* If you have exited the program, sign back in to Mountain View Clinic and select Wilson Metcalf from the patient list.)
- Click on **Policy** to open the office Policy Manual.
- Type "ethics" in the search bar and click on the magnifying glass.

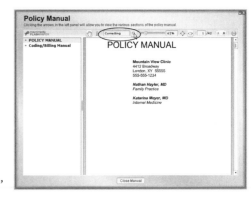

Search for "ethics."

- Read the Work Ethics and Professional Behavior section in the Policy Manual.
- As you answer the following questions, you can leave the Policy Manual open, or if necessary, click **Close Manual** to return to Reception and review the Patient Check-In video again.

1. The Work Ethics and Professional Behavior section in the Policy Manual notes that employees are to show compassion and caring toward patients. Based on these guidelines, describe Kristin's interaction with Mr. Metcalf in the Patient Check-In video.

2. Below, list at least three medical ethics issues and three medical etiquette issues that you can identify from the Patient Check-In video with Mr. Metcalf.

Medical Ethics   **Medical Etiquette**

3. In addition to Kristin's comments about Mr. Metcalf needing soap, what did you notice about her nonverbal communications throughout the video?

Exercise 3

 Writing Activity—Meeting Standards of Medical Ethics and Etiquette

10 minutes

In the previous exercise, you identified breaches of medical ethics and medical etiquette. In this exercise, you will determine the appropriate behaviors and actions that could have avoided these breaches and would satisfy the office policy for professional behavior.

1. When Mr. Metcalf first appeared at Kristin's window to check in, which of the following actions do you think would have demonstrated better medical ethics and etiquette? Select all that apply.

   _____ Ask Mr. Metcalf to supply all his new insurance information immediately.

   _____ Offer Mr. Metcalf a seat before asking for insurance information.

   _____ Ask Mr. Metcalf whether he is in pain and whether he requires assistance.

   _____ Notify a clinical medical assistant immediately that there is a patient in distress in the waiting room.

   _____ Notify the physician about Mr. Metcalf's distress.

   _____ Call 911.

   _____ Insist that Mr. Metcalf complete his new Patient Information Form.

   _____ Close the window to protect yourself from possible infection while making copies of the insurance card.

   _____ Obtain all insurance information after Mr. Metcalf is placed in an examination room.

2. Which of the following actions do you think would have demonstrated better medical ethics and etiquette from the time Mr. Metcalf fell to the floor until the end of the video? Select all that apply.

   _____ Call 911.

   _____ Notify the physician.

   _____ Attempt to help Mr. Metcalf to a chair.

   _____ Use the intercom to call for the red folder and additional assistance.

   _____ Move the other patient in the waiting room away from Mr. Metcalf.

   _____ Quietly document Mr. Metcalf's vital signs.

   _____ Tell Mr. Metcalf that you think he'll be okay.

   _____ Reassure Mr. Metcalf that he will be cared for and that help is on the way.

Exercise 4

  ## CD-ROM Activity—Recognizing the Need for Patient Termination

 20 minutes

- Return to the Reception desk with Wilson Metcalf as your patient. (*Note:* If you have exited the program, sign back in to Mountain View Clinic and select Wilson Metcalf from the patient list.)
- At the Reception desk, click on **Today's Appointments** to review the day's schedule.

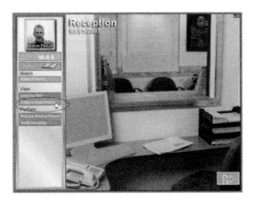

1. What is the name of the patient who has canceled the appointment, and what is the chief complaint?

2. What is the role of the medical assistant in providing information about cancellations to the physician?

→ • Assume that when you obtain the medical record to document the cancellation, you discover that the patient has canceled and rescheduled this appointment three times. He is now 4 weeks late for a return appointment.
- Click **Finish** to close the appointment book and return to the Reception desk.
- Click on **Policy** to open the office Policy Manual.
- Type "cancel" in the search bar and click the magnifying glass to read the office policy regarding canceled appointments.
- Click **Close Manual** to return to the Reception desk.

3. According to the Policy Manual, what is the next step to be taken with this patient who has canceled his last three appointments? Explain your answer.

4. Compose a letter to the above patient, describing the reason for possible termination and the steps needed to remain a patient of Dr. Meyer. The letter should include all of the reasons for possible termination and the need to keep appointments as scheduled. The letter can also state that Dr. Meyer is concerned about continuity of care and the need for patient safety through this continuity of care.

Mountain View Clinic

4412 Broadway / London, XY 55555 / Phone: (555) 555-1234 / Fax (555) 555-1239

Nathan Hayler, MD - Family Practice / Katarina Meyer, MD - Internal Medicine

5. Why does the letter you composed in question 4 need to be certified?

6. After the letter is sent, how much time must be allowed before care is terminated?

Interacting with Patients

Reading Assignment: Chapter 4—Interacting with Patients

Patients: Janet Jones, Jade Wong

Objectives:

- Differentiate between nonverbal and verbal communication.
- Identify factors that can interfere with effective communication.
- Correlate the existence of unmet needs to types of patient behavior in the health care setting.
- Explain the role of empathy in the relationship between the medical assistant and patients.
- Identify importance of sensitivity to cultural differences.

Exercise 1

  CD-ROM Activity—Verbal and Nonverbal Communication

30 minutes

- Sign in to Mountain View Clinic.
- From the patient list, select **Janet Jones**.

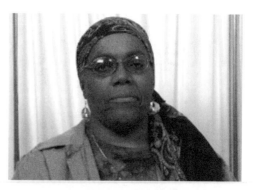

Janet Jones

- On the office map, highlight and click on **Reception**.

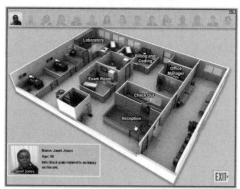

Click on Reception.

- Under the Watch heading, select **Patient Check-In** to view Janet Jones' arrival. Pause the video at the first fade-out.

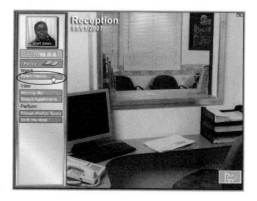

Click on Patient Check-In.

1. What verbal cues does Janet Jones give to Kristin about her mood and condition?

2. What nonverbal cues does Ms. Jones give to Kristin about her mood and condition?

3. What are Kristin's verbal and nonverbal responses to Ms. Jones?

→ • Return to the video and click the play button to watch the rest of the exchange between Kristin and Ms. Jones.

4. In the second half of the video, has there been any change in Ms. Jones' attitude? If yes, describe what you observed and offer a rationale for her attitude change.

5. Has there been any change in Kristin's attitude or response towards Ms. Jones? If yes, describe what you observed and offer a rationale for the change.

6. Below, list at least three things Kristin did well in her communications with Ms. Jones. Then list three or more examples where she could improve in her future communications with patients.

Examples of Good Communication	**Examples of Poor Communication/ Areas for Improvement**

 • Click **Close** to return to the Reception desk.
  • Click the exit arrow and select **Return to Map**.

LESSON 3—INTERACTING WITH PATIENTS **43**

Exercise 2

 CD-ROM Activity—Cultural Differences and Barriers to Communication

15 minutes

- On the office map, select **Jade Wong** as your patient. (*Note:* If you have exited the program, sign back in to Mountain View Clinic and select Jade Wong from the patient list.)

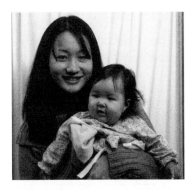

Jade Wong

- Enter the **Exam Room**.

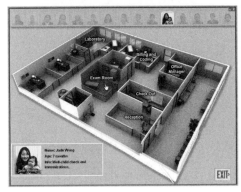

Click on Exam Room.

- Select **Charts** to open Jade's medical record. Review the Patient Information Form.

  1. What is the notation made on the line for Emergency Contact?

→ • Click **Close Chart** to return to the Exam Room. Select **Well-Baby Visit** to watch the video.

  2. Who is the primary communicator for Jade Wong?

3. Who does the medical assistant speak to as she explains the procedure? Is she communicating appropriately with Mr. and Mrs. Wong? Why or why not?

4. The medical assistant in this video needed to overcome a barrier to communication. Listed below are some other potential barriers to communication. For each barrier, offer at least one possible way a medical assistant could overcome the barrier and ensure good communication with the patient.

Barriers to Communication	Recommended Solutions
Patient is deaf or hard of hearing.	
Patient is visually impaired or blind.	
Patient is in a wheelchair.	
Patient has a speech impediment.	

Medical Asepsis and the OSHA Standard

/ᴏᴏ **Reading Assignment:** Chapter 17—Medical Asepsis and the OSHA Standard
  • Microorganisms and Medical Asepsis
  • OSHA Bloodborne Pathogens Standard

Patients: Jean Deere, Louise Parlet, Kevin McKinzie

Objectives:

- Discuss the rationale for handwashing versus hand sanitization.
- Identify the specific circumstances in which handwashing is appropriate.
- Identify the specific circumstances in which hand sanitization is appropriate.
- Examine the policy manual regarding policies of infection control for this office.
- Recognize the circumstances in which the communicability of disease may indicate the use of handwashing versus alcohol-based hand rubs.

Exercise 1

 CD-ROM Activity—Handwashing/Hand Sanitization

 35 minutes

- Sign in to Mountain View Clinic.
- From the patient list, select **Jean Deere**.

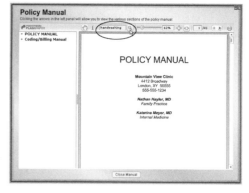

Jean Deere

- On the office map, highlight **Reception** and click to enter the Reception area.

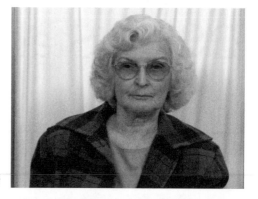

Click on Reception.

- In the Reception area, click on **Policy** to open the Policy Manual.

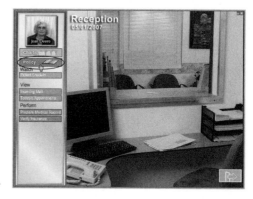

Open the Policy Manual.

- In the Policy Manual search box, type "handwashing" and click on the magnifying glass to search.

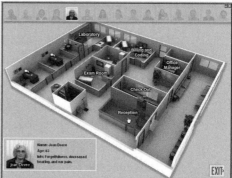

*Type "handwashing" in the search bar
and click on the magnifying glass.*

• Read the section of the Policy Manual on handwashing.

• Go to http://www.cdc.gov/od/oc/media/pressrel/fs021025.htm and read the fact sheet on hand hygiene.

• Click on **Close Manual** when finished. To leave the Reception area, click on the exit arrow in the lower right corner of the screen.

• From the Summary Menu, select **Return to Map**.

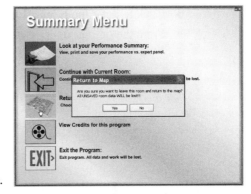

Select Return to Map.

• From the patient list, select **Jesus Santo**, who was the patient seen just before Jean Deere. On the office map, click to enter the **Billing and Coding** area.

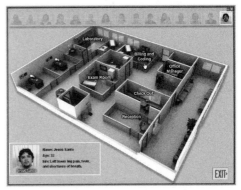

Click on Billing and Coding.

• In the Billing and Coding area, click on **Encounter Form** to review the information for today's visit. Find the diagnosis for Mr. Santo's visit.

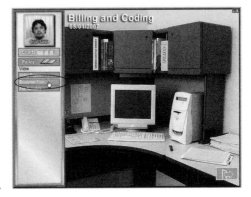

Click on Encounter Form.

1. Based on the diagnosis listed on the Encounter Form for Mr. Santo and your review of the CDC guidelines for hand hygiene, what would be the correct method of hand hygiene to use between patients?

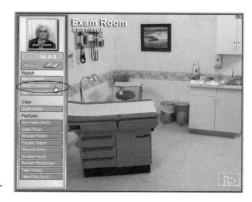

• Click on **Finish** to close the Encounter Form; then click on the exit arrow to leave the Billing and Coding area.

• Click on **Return to Map** and select **Jean Deere** again from the patient list.

• Click to enter the **Exam Room**.

• From the options under Watch, select **Room Preparation** and observe the video.

Click on Room Preparation.

2. Why did the medical assisting extern need to perform handwashing before preparing the room for a patient?

3. According to CDC policy, if the patient seen before Jean Deere did not have a diagnosis with the possibility of disease transmission, what would have been the appropriate form of hand sanitization?

4. _____ True or False: According to the CDC, the use of gloves precludes the need for hand hygiene between patients.

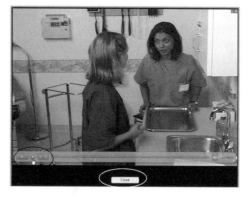

• Either click on the stop button or wait for the video to end; then click on **Close** to return to the Exam Room.

Click on Close to return to the Exam Room.

➤ • From the options under Perform, select **Sanitize Hands** and answer the related question.

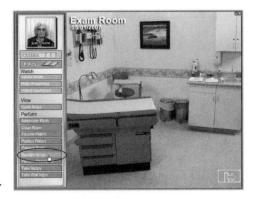

Click on Sanitize Hands.

• Click on **Finish** and then on the exit arrow to leave the Exam Room.
• From the Summary Menu, select **Look at Your Performance Summary** to compare your answers with those of the experts.

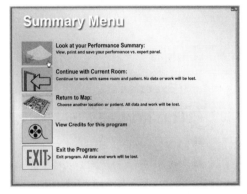

Click on Look at Your Performance Summary.

• Scroll down the Performance Summary to the Sanitize Hands section and check your answer with the experts.
• When you have finished checking your work, click on **Close** and then on **Return to Map**.
• Select **Louise Parlet** from the patient list and click on **Exam Room**.

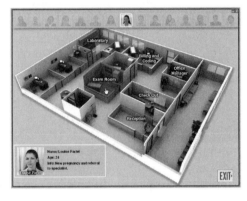

Click on Louise Parlet and then on Exam Room.

• From the Watch menu, select **Infection Control** to watch the video. When the video ends, click **Close**.

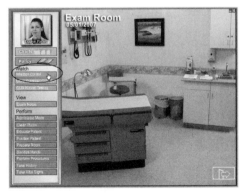

Click on Infection Control.

• Click on the exit arrow and then on **Return to Map**.

5. Would it have been acceptable for the medical assisting extern to clean the table without gloves if she had sanitized her hands prior to and immediately after disposing of the table paper and gown? Why or why not?

6. After the extern has cleaned the examination table and removed gloves, what would be the appropriate means of hand hygiene?

Exercise 2

CD-ROM Activity—Hand Sanitization with Possible Infectious Diseases

🕐 15 minutes

- Select **Kevin McKinzie** from the patient list. (*Note:* If you have exited the program, sign in again to Mountain View Clinic and select Kevin McKinzie from the patient list.)
- On the office map, click on **Check Out**.
- In the **Check Out** area, click on **Charts** and then on the **Patient Medical Information** tab. From the drop-down menu, select **1-Progress Notes** to review today's visit.

Select 1-Progress Notes.

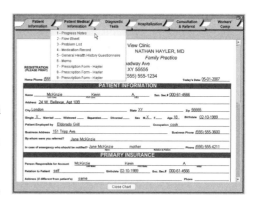

1. What is the possible diagnosis for this patient?

2. With this diagnosis, what would be the safest means of hand hygiene following patient care?

3. _____ According to the CDC, the use of gloves is not necessary when good hand hygiene is used. (True or False)

4. The CDC has recommended the use of alcohol-based hand rubs instead of handwashing in

some instances. Two advantages of hand rubs are that they are _____

and _____.

5. List three times when handwashing is necessary in the medical office.

Regulated Medical Waste

/OⱭ **Reading Assignment:** Chapter 17—Medical Asepsis and the OSHA Standard
  • Regulated Medical Waste

Patients: Shaunti Begay, Hu Huang, Tristan Tsosie

Objectives:

- Recognize what materials are biohazardous.
- Describe the proper disposal of used medical equipment and supplies.
- Identify the proper practice of standard precautions.
- Understand how to apply OSHA standards.
- Discuss the importance of an infection control plan for medical facilities.

Exercise 1

  CD-ROM Activity—Infection Control in the Medical Office Using OSHA Standards

20 minutes

- Sign in to Mountain View Clinic.
- From the patient list, select **Shaunti Begay**.

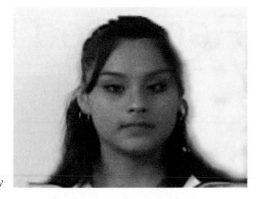

Shaunti Begay

- On the office map, click to enter the **Exam Room**. Inside the Exam Room, click on **Policy** to open the Policy Manual.

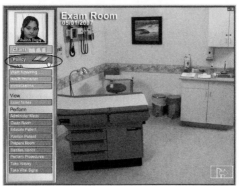

Go to the Exam Room and click on Policy.

- In the Policy Manual search box, type "OSHA" and then click on the magnifying glass to review the relevant section.

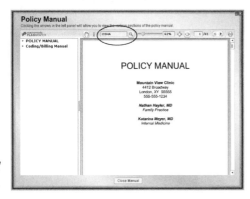

Type "OSHA" and click on the magnifying glass.

- Read the section of the Policy Manual on OSHA Bloodborne Pathogens.

1. Name four body fluids that would be considered biohazardous waste in this medical office.

2. What body secretion is not included in the list of biohazardous waste?

3. What does the term *universal precaution* indicate?

4. What are work practice controls?

5. What are engineering controls?

6. What are PPEs?

7. Does OSHA have any directions for maintaining an examination room? Explain.

• Click on **Close** to exit the Policy Manual.
• Remain in the Exam Room and continue to Exercise 2.

Exercise 2

 CD-ROM Activity—Application of OSHA Standards

 30 minutes

• In this exercise we will continue with Shaunti Begay's visit to the clinic. (*Note:* If you have exited the program, sign in again to Mountain View Clinic, select Shaunti Begay, and go to the Exam Room.)
• From the Exam Room menu, select **Immunization** and watch the video.
• Stop or pause the video at the first fadeout before answering the following questions.

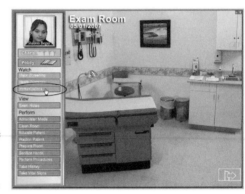

Select Immunization.

1. Did the medical assistant wear the proper PPEs for giving an injection? Explain your answer.

2. Did the medical assistant properly handle the disposal of the gloves and waste from the injection?

3. What engineering controls did you see in the video?

 • Click **Close** to end the video and return to the Exam Room.

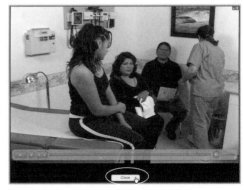

Click on Close.

• Click on the exit arrow to leave the Exam Room.
• From the Summary Menu, select Return to Map.

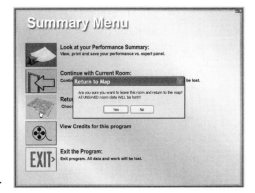

Click on Return to Map.

• Select Hu Huang from the patient list.

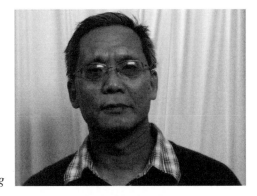

Hu Huang

• Click on Reception on the office map.

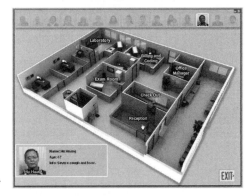

Click on Reception.

• From the Reception area, click on **Patient Check-In** to watch a video of Hu Huang.

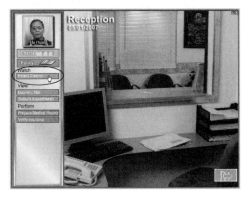

Click on Patient Check-In.

4. Mr. Huang has a productive cough when he approaches the Reception area. He lays a contaminated tissue on the counter just before Kristin takes him to a room. Should she have left the area without disinfecting the counter? Explain your answer.

5. Explain the proper disposal of contaminated tissues.

6. Which of the following are proper steps in infection control that should be observed during the check-in of Mr. Huang? Select all that apply.

_____ Provide tissues as shown in the video.

_____ Allow Mr. Huang to stay in the waiting room.

_____ Throw the tissue in the trash at the desk so that the contamination cannot spread.

_____ Apply gloves before handling the used tissues.

_____ Provide Mr. Huang with a means of disposing of the used tissues in a biohazard waste bag.

_____ Wash hands after disinfecting the counter.

_____ Don a gown and mask when caring for Mr. Huang.

7. Based on the video you watched, how do you think the patients in the waiting room probably felt when the medical assistant stated that Hu Huang might have an infectious disease that could be given to the other patients? Do you think Kristin handled the check-in in an ethical manner? Explain your answer.

8. True or False:

a. _____ Since Mr. Huang laid his contaminated tissue on the counter, OSHA standards would require that Kristin disinfect the counter before allowing another patient to register.

b. _____ Ideally, after Mr. Huang laid his tissue on the counter, Kristin should have donned gloves and removed the tissue before moving the patient to a room.

c. _____ Ideally, in offices where patients may have infectious diseases, a biohazard waste bag should be placed at the check-in window for situations similar to what you saw in the video.

d. _____ Ideally, the check-in desk should have nonsterile gloves available for removing biohazardous waste.

e. _____ Since Kristin did not touch the contaminated tissues, she does not need to sanitize her hands.

f. _____ The better method of sanitization of Kristin's hands would be washing.

• Click **Close** to exit the video and return to the Reception area.
• Click on the exit arrow and then on **Return to Map**.
• Click on **Exam Room** to enter the patient examination area.
• From the Exam Room menu, select **Exam Notes** (under View) and read the documentation for Hu Huang's visit. Click **Finish** when you are finished.

Click on Exam Notes.

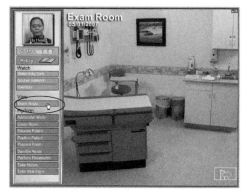

• Now select **Clean Room** (under Perform) and choose the steps that should be taken at the end of Mr. Huang's visit to clean the room before the next patient is seen.
• After making your selections, click **Finish**.
• Click on the exit arrow and select **Look at Your Performance Summary** to check your answers with the experts.

Click on Look at Your Performance Summary.

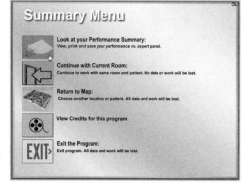

• After reviewing your answers, click **Close** and then **Return to Map** to move on to the next exercise.

Exercise 3

 CD-ROM Activity—Applying Knowledge of Federal Regulations (OSHA)

 15 minutes

- Select **Tristan Tsosie** from the patient list. (*Note:* If you have exited the program, sign in again to Mountain View Clinic and select Trsitan Tsosie from the patient list.)
- Click on **Exam Room** on the office map.
- In the Exam Room, click on **Throat Specimen** and watch the video. Observe the infection control measures.

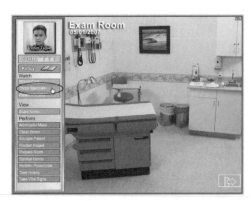

Select Throat Specimen.

1. Which of the following PPEs were used by Cathy when she obtained a throat culture? Select all that apply.

   _____ Sterile gloves

   _____ Nonsterile gloves

   _____ Face shield

   _____ Sterile gown

   _____ Disposable gown

   _____ Goggles

2. True or False:

   a. _____ Cathy followed OSHA policy regarding the PPEs needed for obtaining a throat culture.

   b. _____ The supplies used to collect the throat specimen should be disposed in the biohazard waste container.

   c. _____ The gown and mask may be used again with another patient since Tristan did not cough.

   d. _____ The PPEs used by Cathy must be provided by her.

   e. _____ The biohazard bag is not full at the end of the day, so it is acceptable to add tomorrow's waste and then discard when the bag is full.

   f. _____ Each medical office must have its own infection control system.

   g. _____ Compliance with OSHA standards is required by law.

3. Do you feel that Cathy handled the use of PPEs in an acceptable manner when talking with Tristan? Explain your reasoning.

6

Sterilization and Disinfection

/OꝎ **Reading Assignment:** Chapter 18—Sterilization and Disinfection

Patient: Jose Imero

Objectives:

- Identify the reasons for checking instruments for repairs before wrapping.
- Identify the reasons for performing sanitization before sterilization.
- Discuss the need for double-wrapping some items before sterilization.
- Describe the use of indicator strips in sterilization techniques and quality control.
- Identify the items needed for wrapping articles for sterilization.
- Identify the steps required for wrapping items for sterilization.

Exercise 1

 CD-ROM Activity—Sanitation and Sterilization

 45 minutes

1. What does it mean to *sanitize* equipment?

- Sign in to Mountain View Clinic.
- From the patient list, select **Jose Imero**.

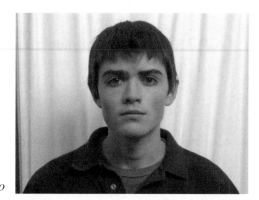

Jose Imero

- On the office map, highlight **Exam Room** and click to enter the patient examination area.

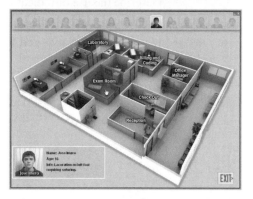

Click on Exam Room.

- In the Exam Room, click on **Sterilization Techniques** and watch the video.

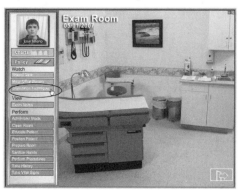

Click on Sterilization Techniques.

2. When do instruments need to be placed in a sanitizing solution?

3. What is the rationale for soaking instruments before sanitization?

4. _____ True or False: Before sanitization, instruments should be rinsed in cool water and dried.

5. Which of the following should be used during sanitization of instruments?
   a. Cold water
   b. Low-sudsing detergent
   c. Brush
   d. Hot water to rinse
   e. All except *a*

6. When articles contain contaminated materials, such as body fluids and blood, which of the following should be used for sanitization?
   a. Cool water
   b. Low-sudsing detergent with neutral pH
   c. Brush
   d. All of the above
   e. All except *a*

7. In the video, Charlie asks Danielle whether she has checked to be sure that the "instruments approximate." What does it mean for an instrument *to approximate*?

8. Why do you think Charlie ask whether the indicator strip was "in date"?

9. What is the reason for the indicator strip?

10. Which of the following supplies are needed when wrapping instruments and equipment for sterilization? Select all that apply.

_____ Wrapping paper or cloth/sterilization pouches

_____ Pencil

_____ Indicator strip or biological sterilization indicator

_____ Pen

_____ Autoclave tape

11. Why should instruments wrapped in paper or cloth be double-wrapped for sterilization?

12. Why is it important to make sure the wrapping material is an appropriate size for the item being wrapped?

13. Charlie told Danielle to begin with the wrapping material in a diamond shape. Why is this important when wrapping articles for sterilization?

14. True or False:

    a. _____ When instruments with movable parts are being wrapped, the joint should be closed to prevent moisture from adhering to the instrument and causing rust.

    b. _____ When instruments with sharp edges are being wrapped, the edges should first be wrapped in gauze.

    c. _____ The sterilization strip shows that the package has been sterilized.

    d. _____ Autoclave tape indicates that the package is sterile.

    e. _____ Any ballpoint pen is acceptable for labeling a package for the autoclave.

    f. _____ The first fold made in wrapping an instrument should be the fold closest to your body at the bottom of the package.

15. Which of the following should appear on the label of a wrapped article for the autoclave? Select all that apply.

    _____ Type of instrument or equipment found in package

    _____ Indicator strip inside

    _____ Date of sterilization

    _____ Initials of person preparing package

    _____ Expiration date for the package

16. Match the columns below to show the correct sequence of steps in wrapping an instrument for autoclaving.

Action	**Order**
_____ Fold the top corner of the wrap toward the center and fold a tab.	a. Step 1
_____ Fold the bottom corner of the wrapping material toward the center and fold a tab.	b. Step 2
_____ Place autoclave tape across the outside corner.	c. Step 3
_____ Flip the instrument in the wrap until it is a neat package.	d. Step 4
_____ Fold each side of the wrap into the center, leaving a tab on each side.	e. Step 5

Vital Signs

/O⯑O **Reading Assignment:** Chapter 19—Vital Signs

Patients: Teresa Hernandez, John R. Simmons

Objectives:

- State the normal range for body temperature.
- Describe conditions that alter body temperature.
- Discuss dangerous levels of body temperature.
- State the normal range for pulse rate.
- Describe conditions that alter the pulse rate and rhythm.
- Discuss pulse rates and rhythms that indicate disease.
- State the normal respiratory rate, depth, and rhythm.
- Describe conditions that alter respiratory function.
- State the normal ranges for blood pressure.
- Describe conditions that alter body pressure, including age-related factors.
- Discuss what is meant by hypertension, prehypertension, and normal blood pressure.

Exercise 1

 CD-ROM Activity—Obtaining Temperature, Pulse, and Respiration

30 minutes

- Sign in to Mountain View Clinic.
- From the patient list, select **Teresa Hernandez**.

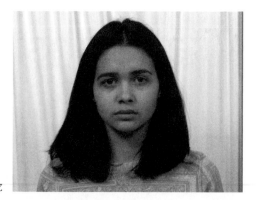

Teresa Hernandez

- On the office map, highlight and click on **Exam Room**.

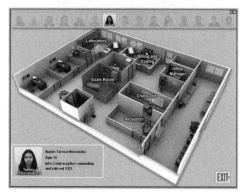

Click on Exam Room.

- Select **Policy** to open the office Policy Manual.

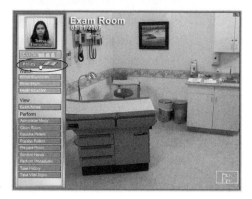

Click on Policy.

- Type "standing orders" in the search bar and click the magnifying glass to read the relevant section.
- When finished, click **Close Manual** to return to the Exam Room.

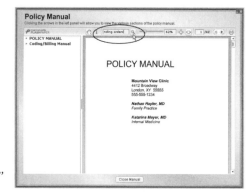

Search for "standing orders."

1. What are the standing order instructions regarding vital signs and physical examinations?

2. Which of the following statements about temperature are true? Select all that apply.

_____ The medical assistant must be aware of the normal ranges of temperature for screening of patient vital signs.

_____ Temperature ranges are the same for all ages.

_____ Equipment used for obtaining temperature readings should be checked on a regular basis for proper working conditions.

_____ All temperature readings have the same baseline, regardless of which site is used to obtain the reading.

_____ Temperature may be taken immediately after a patient eats, smokes, or exercises.

_____ When taking vital signs, the medical assistant should have an organized order in which to obtain the readings.

_____ Usually vital signs are documented in the order of temperature, pulse, and then respirations.

_____ Body temperature is the balance between heat from metabolic processes and the loss of heat from the body.

_____ Normal body temperature ranges are from 97 degrees to 99 degrees Fahrenheit.

_____ Fever is any temperature above 98.6 degrees Fahrenheit.

_____ A temperature of 38 degrees Celsius is considered normal.

3. A body temperature of 98.4 degrees F is considered _____, whereas a

temperature below 97 degrees F is considered _____. If the patient has a

temperature above 100.4 degrees F, it is considered fever, or _____.

4. A person with fever is described as _____, whereas a person without

fever is considered _____.

5. Match each of the following sites with the corresponding normal temperature (or range) for that site.

Temperature (F)	**Site**
_____ 97-99 degrees	a. Axillary
_____ 99.6 degrees	b. Oral
_____ 97.6 degrees	c. Rectal
_____ 98.6 degrees	d. Aural

6. Match each of the following age groups with the corresponding normal temperature (range) and site for that age group.

Age Group	**Temperature (F)/Site**
_____ Newborn	a. 97.6 degrees/axillary
_____ Infant	b. 99.6 degrees/rectal
_____ Child	c. Varies between 97-100 degrees/axillary
_____ Adult	d. 96.8 degrees/oral
_____ Geriatric	e. 98.6 degrees/aural

7. What is specifically being measured when the pulse rate is obtained?

8. Which of the following factors affect the pulse? Select all that apply.

_____ Metabolism

_____ Age

_____ Physical exercise

_____ Emotional states

_____ Gender

_____ Body temperature

_____ Weather conditions

_____ Medications

_____ Respiratory rate

9. Which of the following are sites for obtaining pulse rate? Select all that apply.

_____ Across the abdomen

_____ Popliteal area

_____ Radial and ulnar surfaces

_____ Temporal area

_____ Axillary area

_____ Femoral area

_____ Apically

_____ Brachial area

_____ Carotid areas

_____ Dorsalis pedis

_____ Anterior tibial

10. Match each of the following groups to the corresponding average pulse rate for that group.

Average Pulse Rate	**Group**
_____ 90-140	a. Newborns
_____ 40-60	b. Toddlers
_____ 120-160	c. Children
_____ 65-80	d. School-age children
_____ 60-100	e. Adolescents/adults
_____ 80-110	f. Geriatrics
_____ 75-105	g. Athletes

11. Pulse rates are described by _____, _____, and

_____.

12. What is meant by dysrhythmia?

13. When discussing pulse volume, _____ indicates a fast, weak pulse,

    whereas _____ indicates an extremely full pulse.

14. Why is respiratory rate counted as a vital sign?

15. Which of the following factors affect respirations? Select all that apply.

    _____ Age

    _____ Exercise

    _____ Environment

    _____ Disease processes

    _____ Emotional states

    _____ Gender

    _____ Medications

16. Match each of the following respiratory sounds to its definition.

Sound	**Definition**
_____ Rhonchi	a. High grating sound similar to that of leather pieces rubbing together, heard on auscultation
_____ Wheezes	
_____ Crackles	b. Dry or wet intermittent sound that varies in pitch, similar to the sound of rubbing hair together
_____ Pleural friction rub	c. Deep, low-pitched rumbling sound heard more on expiration
	d. High whistling musical sound heard on both inspiration and expiration

17. Match the following average respiratory rate ranges with the age group to which they apply.

**Average Respiratory
Rate Range**   **Age Group**

_____ 12-20   a. Newborns

_____ 23-35   b. Toddlers

_____ 30-40   c. Children

_____ 18-26   d. School-age children

_____ 20-30   e. Adolescents/Adults

18. The taking in of oxygen is called _____, whereas the breathing out of

carbon dioxide is called _____. Together, these two mechanisms are

considered one _____.

19. Match each of the following terms with its definition.

Definition   **Term**

_____ Dyspnea that is relieved by standing or   a. Apnea
       sitting positions
                                                         b. Sleep apnea
_____ Bluish discoloration of the skin
                                                         c. Adventitious sounds
_____ Difficult breathing
                                                         d. Orthopnea
_____ Absence of respiration
                                                         e. Dyspnea
_____ Abnormal breath sounds
                                                         f. Cyanosis
_____ Absence of respirations during periods of rest

20. True or False:

a. _____ When an aural temperature is taken on a toddler, the auricle should be
              pulled down and back.

b. _____ When an aural temperature is taken on an adult, the auricle should be pulled
              up and back to expose the tympanic membrane.

c. _____ The patient should be told exactly what is being measured when obtaining
              all vital signs.

d. _____ If a pulse rate is being taken, the respiratory rate should be counted at the
              same time.

e. _____ Rectal temperature is a safe procedure for all patients.

f. _____ All patients can have the pulse taken at the radial site.

g. _____ When pulse rates are being recorded, any deviation of rhythm or volume should be documented.

h. _____ When respirations are being recorded, any deviation in rhythm or volume should be documented.

 • From the Exam Room menu, click on **Take Vital Signs** (under the Perform heading).

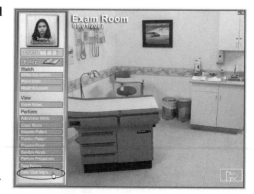

Click on Take Vital Signs.

• As you click on each vital sign, the reading will appear in the corresponding box. Note that there is a check box to mark if the physician needs to be notified of any abnormality.

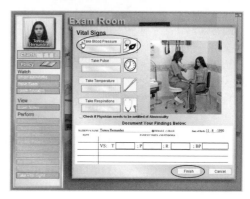

Click each vital sign to get a reading.

• At the bottom of the screen there is room for you to document each vital sign for the patient.
• Record the readings accurately and click **Finish** to return to the Exam Room.

21. Which, if any, of Teresa Hernandez's vital signs are not within normal limits?

 • Click the exit arrow to leave the Exam Room.
• If you like, or if requested by your instructor, you can select **Look at Your Performance Summary** to compare your answers with those of the experts.
• Select **Return to Map** from the Summary Menu.

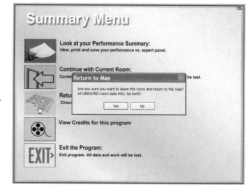

Click on Return to Map.

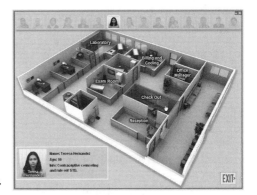

- From the office map, highlight and click on **Check Out** to review the final documentation of Teresa's visit.

Click on Check Out.

- Open **Charts** and select **1-Progress Notes** from the drop-down menu under the **Patient Medical Information** tab.

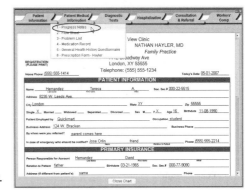

Click on 1-Progress Notes.

- Read the final documentation of Teresa Hernandez's visit.
- Click **Close Chart** to return to the Check Out desk.
- On the Summary Menu, click **Return to Map**.

22. Did the medical assistant obtain the necessary vital signs? Explain your answer.

Exercise 2

 CD-ROM Activity—Obtaining Blood Pressure Readings

 20 minutes

1. What is specifically assessed by blood pressure measurements?

2. Why is the diastolic pressure always above zero?

3. Match each of the following terms with its definition.

Term	**Definition**
_____ Hypertension	a. Pressure on the walls of the arteries when the heart is at rest
_____ Pulse pressure	b. Blood pressure over 140/90
_____ Systolic pressure	c. Blood pressure below 90/60
_____ Hypotension	d. Pressure on the walls of the arteries when the heart is contracting
_____ Diastolic pressure	e. The difference between systolic and diastolic pressure

4. Which of the following factors affect blood pressure? Select all that apply.

_____ Time of day

_____ Age

_____ Environment

_____ Exercise

_____ Gender

_____ Emotions

_____ Body position

_____ Amount of sleep

_____ Medications

5. Define normal blood pressure, prehypertensive state, and hypertension.

6. What is the difference between stage 1 hypertension and stage 2 hypertension?

7. The equipment needed for obtaining blood pressure includes a _____

   and _____.

8. Blood pressure cuffs come in the following sizes: _____,

   _____, and _____.

9. The sounds heard as blood pressure is being taken are called _____.

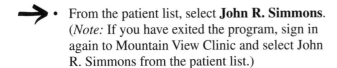 • From the patient list, select **John R. Simmons**.
   (*Note:* If you have exited the program, sign in
   again to Mountain View Clinic and select John
   R. Simmons from the patient list.)

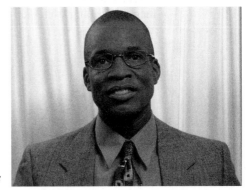

John R. Simmons

• On the office map, click on **Check Out**.
• Click on **Charts** and select **1-Progress Notes** from the drop-down menu under the **Patient Medical Information** tab.
• Read the final documentation of Dr. Simmons' visit.

10. Which, if any, of the vital signs for Dr. Simmons are not within normal limits?

11. According to American Heart Association standards, what is the interpretation of the blood pressure readings taken by the medical assistant?

12. The blood pressure readings for Dr. Simmons are higher when taken the second time. What is a logical explanation for the difference?

13. Why do you think Dr. Meyer wants Dr. Simmons to take blood pressure readings at home and record them?

14. Notice that Dr. Simmons' blood pressure reading taken from the left arm is more elevated than the reading from the right arm. What is an explanation for this?

Exercise 3

Writing Activity—Documentation of Vital Signs

10 minutes

1. Using today's date and time, accurately document the following scenario on the form below:

Judy Marks, age 69 (born 4-27-38), is taking medication for hypertensive disease and is seen at the office on a regular basis. Today she has come in to have her vital signs checked by the medical assistant. Her pulse is 104, weak, and difficult to obtain, with a skipped beat every six beats. Her rate of breathing is 24 times a minute but shallow. Her temperature is 97.6 degrees. Blood pressure is 176/104 in the left arm and 170/102 in the right arm.

PATIENT'S NAME _Judy Marks_ ☒ FEMALE ☐ MALE	Date of Birth: _04/27/38_

DATE	PATIENT VISITS AND FINDINGS

ALLERGIC TO _____

PAGE ____ of ____

ORDER #25-7138-01 • © 1999 BIBBERO SYSTEMS, INC • PETALUMA, CA   TO REORDER CALL 800-BIBBERO (800-242-2376) OR FAX (800) 242-9330 MFG IN USA

2. Which, if any, of the findings on the form in the previous question need to be reported to the physician before Judy Marks leaves the office? Which are abnormal?

Preparing for the Physical Examination

Reading Assignment: Chapter 20—The Physical Examination

Patients: Jean Deere, Louise Parlet

Objectives:

- Describe the steps necessary in preparing an examination room for patient care.
- List supplies needed for a complete physical examination.
- Describe the steps necessary in cleaning the examination or treatment room following patient care.

Exercise 1

  CD-ROM Activity—Preparing Examination or Treatment Room for Patient Care

⏱ 30 minutes

- Sign in to Mountain View Clinic.
- From the patient list, select **Jean Deere**.

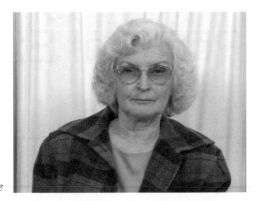

Jean Deere

- On the office map, highlight and click on **Exam Room**.

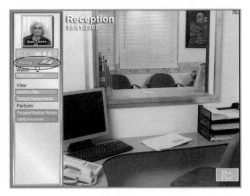

Click on Exam Room.

- Click on **Policy** to open the office Policy Manual.

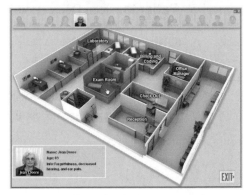

Click on Policy.

- In the search bar type "room maintenance" and click on the magnifying glass.

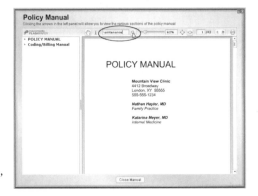

Search for "room maintenance."

- Read the office policy for the preparation of examination/treatment rooms.
- Click **Close Manual** to return to the Exam Room.
- Under the Watch heading, select **Room Preparation** to view the video.

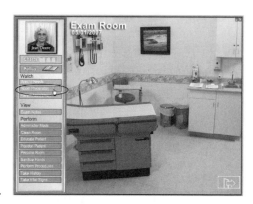

Click on Room Preparation.

- At the end of the video, click **Close** to return to the Exam Room.

1. The medical assisting extern washed her hands before setting up the examination/treatment room. Why is this an important step in room preparation?

2. The medical assistant extern asked Armeeta about Ms. Deere's symptoms. Why is this information important when preparing a room for the patient?

3. True or False:

   a. _____ Infection control is important when preparing a room for a patient.

   b. _____ When preparing the room for a physical examination, the medical assistant should prepare all of the available equipment so that the physician can make a decision about what is needed.

   c. _____ The general cleanliness of the room has nothing to do with the patient's feelings about the entire medical office.

   d. _____ Waste receptacles in the examination/treatment room should be emptied frequently.

   e. _____ Biohazardous receptacles should be changed after any patient care that involves gross biohazard waste.

   f. _____ Sharps biohazard containers should be emptied daily.

   g. _____ Equipment for the examination should be placed at easy access for the physician and, if possible, in the order of use.

h. _____ The medical assistant should know how to operate and care for the equipment found in examination and treatment rooms.

i. _____ The room temperature should be determined by what is comfortable for the physician.

j. _____ All equipment in the examination room should be disposable.

k. _____ Proper disposal of equipment following use is an important factor in infection control.

l. _____ Improperly checked equipment and supplies may cause injury to a patient.

4. Match each of the following pieces of equipment to its description or purpose

Equipment	Description or Purpose
_____ Sphygmomanometer	a. Light on movable stand
_____ Drape	b. Covering to reduce patient exposure
_____ Patient gown	c. Used to test neurological reflexes
_____ Thermometer	d. Long stick with cotton cover used to obtain specimens or to cleanse an area when dampened
_____ Cotton-tipped applicator	e. Small flashlight used to check pupils
_____ Tongue depressor	f. Instrument used to check hearing
_____ Lubricant	g. Instrument used to measure blood pressure
_____ Tape measure	h. Instrument used to measure temperature
_____ Tuning fork	i. Instrument used to auscultate sounds
_____ Percussion hammer	j. Device used to measure parts of the body
_____ Speculum	k. Covering for hands for good infection control practices
_____ Ophthalmoscope	l. Covering with sleeves to provide modesty and warmth for the patient
_____ Otoscope	m. Smooth wooden blade used to examine mouth and throat
_____ Stethoscope	n. Instrument used to examine eyes
_____ Penlight	o. Instrument used to open a body orifice
_____ Gooseneck lamp	p. Instrument used to examine ear canal
_____ Disposable gloves	q. Agent used to reduce friction

→ • Click on **Exam Notes** to open the physician's notes on Ms. Deere for this visit. When finished reading, click **Finish** to return to the Exam Room.

5. Armeeta was correct in assuming Dr. Meyer would want to do an ear lavage and a pulse oximeter reading. What additional test did Dr. Meyer want done at this visit?

• Under the Perform heading, select **Prepare Room**.

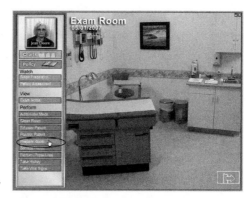

Select Prepare Room.

• Select the first item needed for Ms. Deere's visit from the Available Supplies list and click **Add Item** to confirm your choice. The items you select will appear in the Selected Supplies box.

• Repeat this step until you are satisfied you have everything you need from the list. (*Note:* The Exam Notes are available if you need to refer to them.)

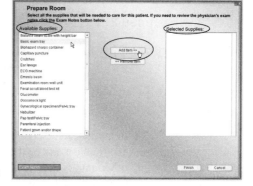

Select the supplies needed for this visit.

• After making all your selections, click **Finish** to return to the Exam Room.

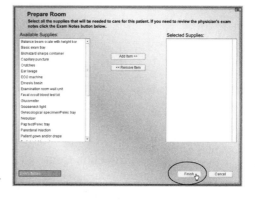

Click Finish to return to the Exam Room.

- Click the exit arrow to go to the Summary Menu.
- Click on **Look at Your Performance Summary**. Scroll down to the Prepare Room section to compare your answers with those of the experts. This summary can also be printed or saved for your instructor.

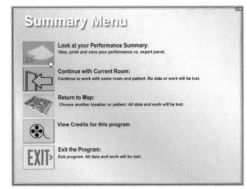

Click on Look at Your Performance Summary.

- Click on **Close** to return to the Summary Menu.
- Click on **Return to Map** and continue to the next exercise.

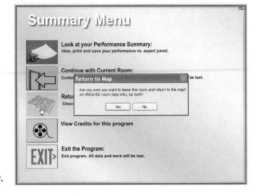

Click on Return to Map.

Exercise 2

 CD-ROM Activity—Maintaining the Examination or Treatment Room Following Patient Care

 30 minutes

- From the patient list, select **Louise Parlet**. (*Note:* If you have exited the program, sign in again to Mountain View Clinic and select Louise Parlet from the patient list.)

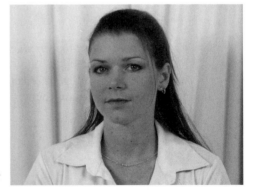

Louise Parlet

- On the office map, highlight and click on **Exam Room**.
- Select **Infection Control** (under Watch) and view the video. At the end of the video, click **Close** to return to the Exam Room.
- Next, click on **Policy** to open the Policy Manual.
- In the search bar, type "room maintenance" and click on the magnifying glass to review.

1. What does the Policy Manual indicate should be performed after each patient has been seen?

2. During the video, did the medical assistant follow the Policy Manual while cleaning the room? Explain your answer.

3. During the video, did you see a break in infection control by the medical assisting extern? Explain.

4. True or False:

   a. _____ The medical assistant should use gloves, gown, and face shield when cleaning the examination room after a patient.

   b. _____ The medical assistant should disinfect the table, supply tray, and counter/table tops after each patient.

   c. _____ The nondisposable supplies and equipment should be disinfected and properly stored when cleaning the room.

   d. _____ Nondisposable equipment should be sanitized and sterilized as necessary before storage.

   e. _____ The office Policy Manual contains all information needed for the correct cleaning of a room following a patient exam.

   f. _____ The physician will inform the medical assistant of the items that must be discarded and those that should be sanitized and used again.

   g. _____ Items such as ophthalmoscopes, otoscopes, and tuning forks do not require sanitization following use in patient care.

   h. _____ Standard precautions should be followed when preparing and cleaning the examination/treatment room.

i. _____ If the medical assistant does not have time between patients to completely clean the room, it is more important to keep the appointment schedule on time than to clean the room.

j. _____ It is permissible for the medical assistant to clean a room after the following patient has been placed in the examination/treatment room.

k. _____ Teamwork is essential in keeping the office neat, clean, and ready for patients.

The Physical Examination

∕☯ **Reading Assignment:** Chapter 20—The Physical Examination

Patients: Teresa Hernandez, Jean Deere

Objectives:

- List the information needed to prepare the patient for a physical examination.
- Use the Policy Manual in preparing the patient for a physical examination.
- Discuss legal and ethical boundaries when preparing a patient for a physical examination.
- Describe the positions used for physical examinations and the indications for each.
- Describe the ethical role of the medical assistant when assisting with a physical examination.
- Discuss patient safety measures during a physical examination.
- Describe the importance of efficiency when assisting the examiner.

Exercise 1

CD-ROM Activity—Preparing an Established Patient for Physical Examination

20 minutes

- Sign in to Mountain View Clinic.
- From the patient list, select **Jean Deere**.

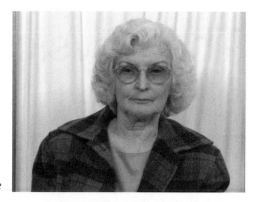

Jean Deere

- On the office map, highlight and click on **Exam Room**.

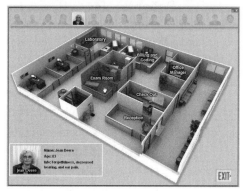

Click on Exam Room.

- Under the Watch heading, select **Patient Assessment** to view the video.
- At the end of the video, click **Close** to return to the Exam Room.
- Click on **Policy** to open the office Policy Manual. Type "standing orders" in the search bar.

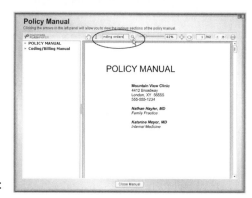

Type "standing orders" in the search bar.

- Click on the magnifying glass and read the Standing Orders section (pages 23-26).
- Click **Close Manual** to return to the Exam Room.

1. What clothing should be removed for Ms. Deere's physical examination?

2. What supplies should Armeeta be sure are available on the table to assist Ms. Deere's son James in preparing his mother for exam?

3. Armeeta has allowed Ms. Deere's son to assist with disrobing. Is that appropriate? Why or why not?

4. When would it not be appropriate to allow or suggest that a family member help disrobe a patient?

5. Why is it important for Armeeta to offer to help Ms. Deere onto the table?

6. For safety reasons, when should Ms. Deere be positioned on the exam table?

7. Is it acceptable to leave the room when a confused, debilitated, or geriatric patient is on the exam table? Why or why not?

8. What position would be appropriate for placing Ms. Deere on the exam table?

- Click the exit arrow to leave the Exam Room.
- From the Summary Menu, click on **Return to Map** and continue to the next exercise.

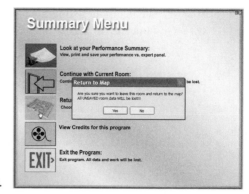

Click on Return to Map.

Exercise 2

 CD-ROM Activity—Preparing a Young Adult and Assisting with a Routine Physical Examination

 20 minutes

- From the patient list, select **Teresa Hernandez**. (*Note:* If you have exited the program, sign in again to Mountain View Clinic and select Teresa Hernandez from the patient list.)

Teresa Hernandez

- On the office map, highlight and click on **Reception**.

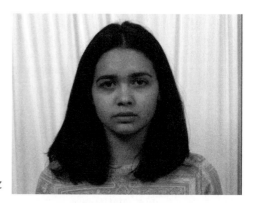

Click on Reception.

- Click on **Today's Appointments** to view the schedule. On the schedule find the reason for Teresa Hernandez's visit.

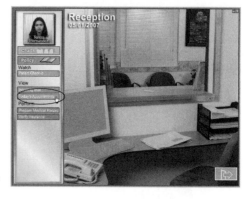

Click on Today's Appointments.

- Click **Finish** to close the appointment book and return to the Reception desk.
- If you wish, you may also review the Policy Manual section on Standing Orders once more before answering the following questions.

1. What is the reason for Teresa's appointment, and what is her status in the medical office that will affect the physical exam preparations?

2. What preliminary steps must the clinical medical assistant complete before a physical examination?

3. What clothing should Teresa remove for her examination?

- Click on the exit arrow to leave Reception.
- From the Summary Menu, click **Return to Map**.
- On the office map, highlight and click on **Exam Room**.
- Select **Ethical Boundaries** (under Watch) to view the video. At the end of the video, click **Close** to return to the Exam Room.

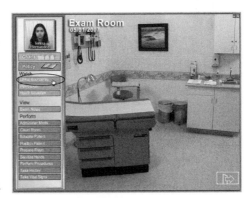

Select Ethical Boundaries.

4. Teresa appeared to be very nervous and uneasy about discussing her chief complaint. What do you think of the way that Armeeta, the medical assistant, handled the situation?

5. Because of the privacy issues surrounding contraception, especially with a teenage patient, Armeeta was faced with ethical and confidentiality boundaries in preparing Teresa to talk with the physician. Do you think that Armeeta provided the guidance needed to place Teresa more at ease? Explain your answer.

6. Would it have been appropriate for Armeeta to tell Teresa that what is said in the office is confidential? Why or why not?

7. Armeeta explained to Teresa to completely disrobe and to put on the gown, but can you identify any important information that she did not included in her instructions?

→ • Under Watch, select and view the next video, **Pelvic Exam**.

8. In the video, what are the ways that Armeeta assists Dr. Hayler? Select all that apply.

_____ Passes instruments

_____ Takes instruments after use

_____ Waits for Dr. Hayler to ask for instruments

_____ Is prepared to give Dr. Hayler needed supplies promptly

_____ Explains the procedure and the need for infection control

_____ Disposes of Dr. Hayler's disposable equipment

_____ Asks Dr. Hayler to dispose of equipment

_____ Has prepared tray and passes all supplies on the tray for use

_____ Has supplies prepared that might be used for a pelvic exam

_____ Accepts specimen for laboratory testing

_____ Prepares label for specimen transport

_____ Has gooseneck lamp adjusted for proper lighting of area being examined

_____ Has patient in proper position for a pelvic examination

9. How did Armeeta provide safety measures for Teresa?

10. Why is it important for Armeeta to have all supplies and equipment available for the physician and to efficiently hand these to the physician without his asking?

11. Teresa is in the _____ position.

Measuring Height and Weight

Reading Assignment: Chapter 20—The Physical Examination
- Height and Weight

Patients: Shaunti Begay, Jean Deere

Objectives:

- Describe the correct methodology for measuring height on an adult.
- Describe the correct methodology for measuring weight on an adult.
- Convert height from inches to feet and inches.
- Convert height and weight from metric to English measurements.
- Convert height and weight from English to metric measurements.
- State the importance of measuring height and weight on each office visit.

Exercise 1

  CD-ROM Activity—Measuring Height

15 minutes

- Sign in to Mountain View Clinic.
- From the patient list, select **Shaunti Begay**.

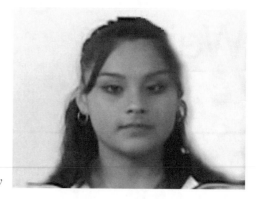

Shaunti Begay

- On the office map, highlight and click on **Exam Room**.

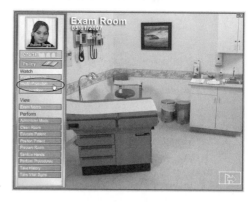

Click on Exam Room.

- Under the Watch heading, select **Health Promotion** to view the video.

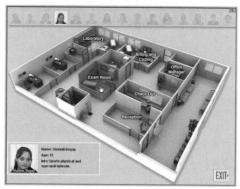

Click on Health Promotion.

- Using the control buttons at the bottom of the video screen, stop the video at the first fade-out.

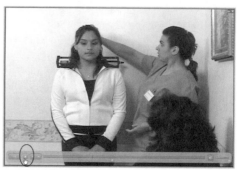

Stop the video at the first fade-out.

- Click **Close** to return to the Exam Room.

1. Why should Shaunti remove her shoes before her height and weight are measured?

2. Why is it important to measure a child's height at each office visit through adolescence?

3. Why is it important to measure all adults with each office visit after the age of 60?

4. Shaunti is wearing socks. If she were not wearing socks, what would have been the appropriate action by the medical assistant before having her stand on the scale?

5. What is the correct angle of the head bar when measuring height?

6. The height measurements on medical scales are marked in _____-inch increments.

7. The medical assistant stated that Shaunti is 5 feet 2 inches tall, which would be _____ inches.

- Click the exit arrow at the bottom right of the screen to leave the Exam Room.
- From the Summary Menu, click **Return to Map**.

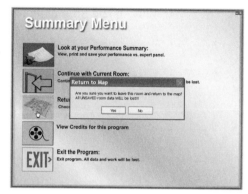

Click on Return to Map.

Exercise 2

 CD-ROM Activity—Measuring Weight

 15 minutes

1. How is quality control performed on scales?

2. What safety steps does the medical assistant need to take with all patients when measuring weight?

3. What weight calibration marking is used on most standing scales found in medical offices?

- From the patient list, select **Jean Deere**. (*Note:* If you have exited the program, sign in again to Mountain View Clinic and select Jean Deere from the patient list.)

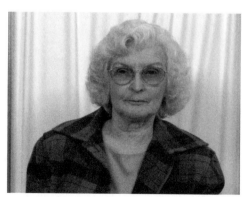

Jean Deere

- On the office map, highlight and click on **Exam Room**.
- Under the Watch heading, select **Patient Assessment** to view the video.

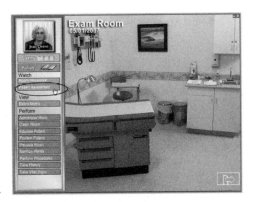

Click on Patient Assessment.

- At the end of the video, click **Close** to return to the Exam Room.

4. Did the medical assistant handle Ms. Deere appropriately to obtain an accurate measurement of the patient's weight?

5. The medical assistant offered to help Ms. Deere to the scales. Why would this be so important with this patient?

6. Notice the placement of the walker over the scales. Why is this important to help in supporting Ms. Deere? When a walker is used in this way, what observations must the medical assistant make to ensure an accurate reading?

7. Ms. Deere is confused, and her son thinks she might have early Alzheimer disease. Do you think that the medical assistant was professional and appropriate in her handling of the patient? Explain your answer. Was it appropriate for Ms. Deere's son to be with her during the weight measurement? Why or why not?

➔ • In the Exam Room, click on **Charts** and select **1-Progress Notes** from the drop-down menu under the **Patient Medical Information** tab.

8. Based on the Progress Notes, what was Jean Deere's weight on her last visit on 9-21-06?

9. Ms. Deere's weight on this visit is 120 pounds. Do you see a reason for the medical assistant to ask questions about her eating habits while taking the health history? Explain.

➔ • Click **Close Chart** to return to the Exam Room.
   • Click on **Policy** to open the office Policy Manual.

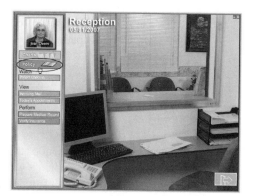

Click on Policy.

• In the search bar, type "standing orders" and click on the magnifying glass to read the relevant section of the manual.

10. Did the medical assistants follow the correct protocol for Shaunti Begay and Jean Deere, according to what you read in the Policy Manual? Explain your answer.

Exercise 3

Writing Activity—Conversions for Mensuration

15 minutes

Use the formulas provided below to calculate answers to the questions in this exercise.

- Weight conversion of kilograms to pounds: Multiply kilograms by 2.2 (1 kg = 2.2 lb).
- Weight conversion of pounds to kilograms: Divide kilograms by 2.2 (2.2 lb = 1 kg).
- Height conversion of inches to feet and inches: Divide the total number of inches by 12; then express the remainder as inches (12 in = 1 ft).
- Height conversion of inches to centimeters: Multiply inches by 2.5 (1 in = 2.5 cm).
- Height conversion of centimeters to inches: Divide centimeters by 2.5 (2.5 cm = 1 in).

1. Joan Neiman weighs 64 kilograms. What is her weight in pounds?

2. Shaunti Begay is 5 feet 2 inches tall. What is her height in centimeters?

3. Jean Deere weighs 120 pounds. What is her weight in kilograms?

4. Sara McHugh is 68 inches tall. What is her height in feet and inches?

5. Isaiah Franklin is 185 centimeters tall. What is his height in inches? In feet and inches?

Eye and Ear Assessment

Reading Assignment: Chapter 21—Eye and Ear Assessment and Procedures

Patients: Shaunti Begay, Jean Deere

Objectives:

- Define visual acuity.
- Differentiate the skills and responsibilities of an ophthalmologist, optometrist, and optician.
- Explain the significance of the top and bottom numbers next to each line of letters on the Snellen Eye Chart.
- Identify conditions that may cause conductive and sensorineural hearing loss.
- List and describe the ways in which hearing acuity can be tested.

Exercise 1

 CD-ROM Activity—The Eye Exam

 15 minutes

- Sign in to Mountain View Clinic.
- From the patient list, select **Shaunti Begay**.

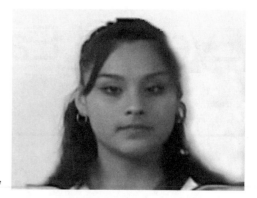

Shaunti Begay

- On the office map, highlight and click on **Exam Room**.

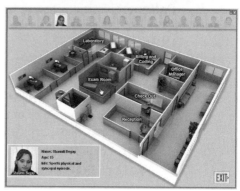

Click on Exam Room.

- Under the Watch heading, select **Vision Screening** to view the video.
- Click **Close** to return to the Exam Room.

1. The test Lisa is about to administer to Shaunti will assess her _____.

2. Lisa instructs Shaunti to cover one eye with the _____.

3. Lisa also shows Shaunti what she will need to read for this screening. The tool shown in the video used to measure distance vision is called the _____.

4. Shaunti is told to stand on a specific spot before beginning the test. This spot should measure a distance of _____ from the chart.

5. Why does Shaunti need to cover one eye as she reads the chart?

6. Shaunti's mother is a very active participant during Shaunti's visit. In addition to speaking for Shaunti, she is also standing very close to her during the eye exam. Is this appropriate? Why or why not?

• In the Exam Room, click the exit arrow and select **Return to Map**.

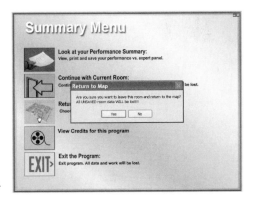

Click on Return to Map.

• On the office map, select **Check Out** and click to enter.

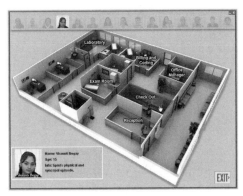

Click on Check Out.

• Click on **Charts** to open Shaunti's medical record.

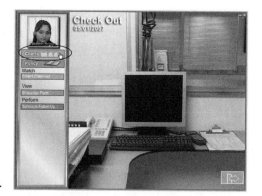

Click on Charts.

• From under the **Patient Medical Information** tab, select **2-Progress Notes** to review the documentation of Shaunti's visit.

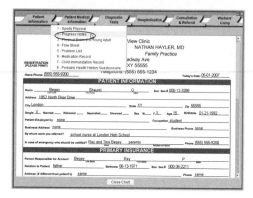

Click on 2-Progress Notes.

7. Scroll up to the first entry and read the results of Shaunti's vision screening. Will Shaunti need corrective lenses?

• Click the exit arrow at the bottom right of the screen to leave the Check Out area.
• From the Summary Menu, click **Return to Map**.

Exercise 2

 CD-ROM Activity—Examining the Ear

 15 minutes

- From the patient list, select **Jean Deere**.
  (*Note:* If you have exited the program, sign in
  again to Mountain View Clinic and select Jean
  Deere from the patient list.)

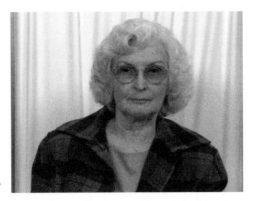

Jean Deere

- On the office map, highlight and click on **Exam Room**.
- In the Exam Room, select **Exam Notes** to review the doctor's documentation of Ms. Deere's
  exam.

1. Dr. Hayler noted Ms. Deere's exam was unremarkable except for what finding?

2. What tests were administered to Ms. Deere relative to this finding? What were the results?

3. The _____ compares the duration of sound perception by air conduction with that of bone conduction.

4. The _____ helps determine whether a patient hears better in one
   ear than the other.

5. Based on the test results and the findings documented by Dr. Hayler, Ms. Deere has what
   type of hearing loss?

6. What treatment did Ms. Deere receive for this problem? What effect should this have on her symptoms?

7. What should be added to Ms. Deere's ear before irrigating it with water? Why?

12

Physical Agents to Promote Tissue Healing

📖 **Reading Assignment:** Chapter 22—Physical Agents to Promote Tissue Healing

Patients: Tristan Tsosie, Janet Jones, Jose Imero

Objectives:

- Identify examples of moist and dry applications of heat and cold.
- State the factors to consider when applying heat and cold.
- List the effects of local application of heat and the reasons for applying heat.
- List the effects of local application of cold and the reasons for applying cold.
- List factors that are taken into consideration when ambulatory aids are prescribed.

Exercise 1

 CD-ROM Activity—Application of Heat and Cold

 15 minutes

- Sign in to Mountain View Clinic.
- From the patient list, select **Tristan Tsosie**.

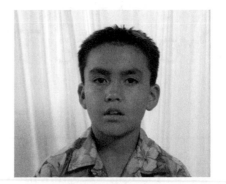

Tristan Tsosie

- On the office map, highlight and click on
  Exam Room.

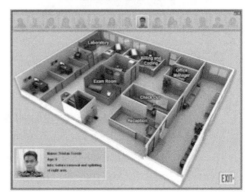

Click on Exam Room.

- Under the **Consultation and Referral** tab, select **1-Consultation Notes**.
- Read the documentation for Tristan's orthopedic consultation.

1. Why was Tristan being seen by the orthopedic surgeon?

2. Scroll through the report and read the results of Tristan's x-ray under the Imaging heading. What are the results?

3. What is the plan for Tristan documented at the end of the report?

4. The application of ice is an example of:
    a. dry cold.
    b. cold compress.
    c. moist cold.
    d. chemical cold.

5. Which of the following are valid reasons why ice should be applied in Tristan's case? Select all that apply.

    _____   To reduce swelling

    _____   To keep the bones in one place

    _____   To reduce pain

    _____   To slow bleeding

    _____   To reduce the chance of infection

    _____   To keep Tristan distracted from his pain

➡ • Click **Close Chart** to return to the Exam Room.
  • Click the exit arrow and select **Return to Map**.

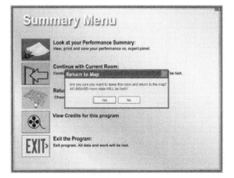

Click on Return to Map.

• On the office map, select **Janet Jones**.

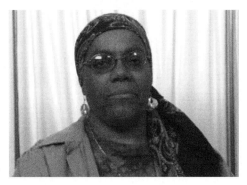

Janet Jones

• Highlight and click on the **Exam Room** to enter.

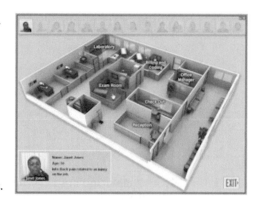

Click on Exam Room.

• Click on **Exam Notes** to open the documentation of Ms. Jones' exam.

6. What is the reason for Ms. Jones' visit?

7. What type of treatment has Ms. Jones tried before coming to the office to see the doctor?

8. The application of a heating pad is an example of:
   a. hot compress.
   b. moist heat.
   c. dry heat.
   d. chemical heat.

9. What are some of the benefits of applying heat in Ms. Jones' case?

10. Ms. Jones' back pain was the result of a fall, which might have strained or sprained her back. Was heat the most appropriate treatment in this case?

• Click **Finish** to close the Exam Notes.
 • Click the exit arrow at the bottom right of the screen.
 • From the Summary Menu, click **Return to Map**.

 Exercise 2

 CD-ROM Activity—Ambulatory Aids

15 minutes

 • From the patient list, select **Jose Imero**. (*Note:* If you have exited the program, sign back in to Mountain View Clinic and select Jose Imero from the patient list.)

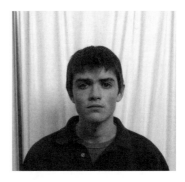

Jose Imero

 • On the office map, highlight and click on **Exam Room**.
 • Select **Exam Notes** from the menu and read the documentation of Jose's visit.

 1. What is the reason for Jose's visit?

 2. What is the plan for Jose's treatment?

 • Click **Finish** to close the Exam Notes.
 • Under the Watch heading, select **Minor Office Surgery** to view the video.
 • At the end of the video, click **Close** to return to the Exam Room.

3. Charlie, the medical assistant, was fitting Jose with what type of crutches?

4. Charlie believes the crutches are too short and wants to adjust them for Jose's height. What problems could Jose encounter if the crutches are left too short?

5. After Charlie adjusts the crutches, what should he have Jose do before leaving the office? Why?

The Gynecologic Examination and Prenatal Care

Oᴍᴅ **Reading Assignment:** Chapter 23—The Gynecologic Examination and Prenatal Care

Patients: Renee Anderson, Louise Parlet

Objectives:

- Obtain the necessary information for gynecologic and prenatal examinations.
- Discuss the legal and ethical boundaries of preparing a patient for a gynecologic/prenatal examination.
- Discuss the legal and ethical boundaries associated with domestic abuse.
- Describe the importance of efficiency when assisting with physical examinations.
- Identify the specific patient history information that is needed for a prenatal examination.
- Plan how a medical assistant should handle domestic abuse concerns ethically and professionally.
- Assess how verbal and nonverbal communications are used with domestic abuse.

Exercise 1

  CD-ROM Activity—Assisting with a Prenatal Examination

45 minutes

- Sign in to Mountain View Clinic.
- From the patient list, select **Louise Parlet**.

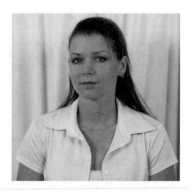

Louise Parlet

- On the office map, highlight and click on **Exam Room**.

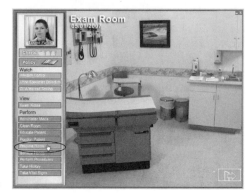

Click on Exam Room.

- In the Exam Room, click on **Exam Notes** to view the documentation for Ms. Parlet's visit.

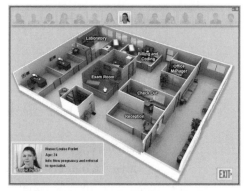

Click on Exam Notes.

- Click **Finish** to close the Exam Notes and return to the Exam Room.
- Under the Perform heading, click **Prepare Room** to select the supplies needed for Ms. Parlet's visit. (*Note:* You can reopen the Exam Notes for reference as you make your selections.)

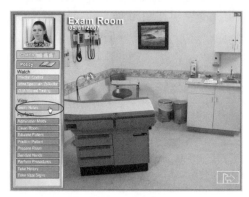

Click on Prepare Room.

- From the alphabetical list of Available Supplies, select the first item needed for Ms. Parlet's visit and click **Add Item** to confirm your choice. The items you select will appear in the Selected Supplies column.

- Repeat this step until you are satisfied you have everything you need from the list.

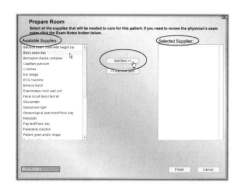

Select the supplies needed for this visit.

- Do NOT close this window. Keep the Prepare Room wizard open as you continue with the lesson.

1. Match the columns below to indicate the order in which the items will be needed for a gynecologic examination.

Order of Use	Item
_____ First	a. Water-soluble lubricant
_____ Second	b. Cotton swabs
_____ Third	c. Lab requisition
_____ Fourth	d. Gloves for physician
_____ Fifth	e. Speculum
_____ Sixth	f. Gloves for medical assistant
_____ Seventh	g. Culture transport, if applicable

- Using the open Prepare Room wizard, confirm that you have chosen the necessary supplies for Louise Parlet's Pap smear. When you click on an item, a photo of that item will appear, which can be used for reference as you review your list of supplies.

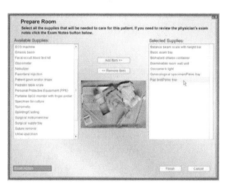

A photo of each item selected is available for reference.

2. Match the columns below to indicate the order in which the supplies will be needed for the Pap smear procedure.

Order of Use	Item
_____ First	a. Glass slides or specimen preservative
_____ Second	b. Lubricant for rectal examination
_____ Third	c. Fixative for slides
_____ Fourth	d. Permanent marker for marking Pap smear slides
_____ Fifth	e. Pen for completing lab request form
_____ Sixth	f. Cervical brush or applicators for obtaining Pap specimen
_____ Seventh	g. Lab requisition form

⮕ • After completing all the selections you wish to make in the Prepare Room wizard, click **Finish** to return to the Exam Room.

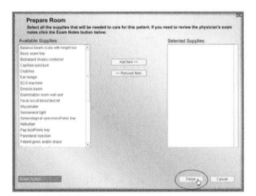

Click Finish to Return to Exam Room.

• Remain in the Exam Room with Ms. Parlet. Under the Perform heading, click on **Position Patient**.

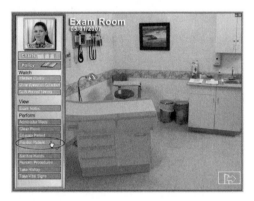

Click on Position Patient.

• Select all positions Louise Parlet will be placed in during her exam.
• Click **Finish** to return to the Exam Room.

3. List the positions that will be used for Ms. Parlet's exam in the order in which they should occur.

4. Explain the use of each of the positions you listed in the previous question.

 • Remain in the Exam Room with Ms. Parlet.
   • Click on **Perform Procedures** and review the list of possible procedures.

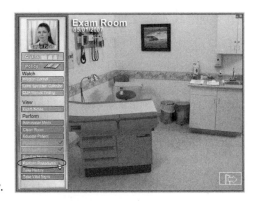

Click on Perform Procedures.

• Select all procedures that should be performed on Louise Parlet during her visit. (*Remember:* You can click on **Exam Notes** to reopen and review these notes as needed to make your selections.)
• Click **Finish** to return to the Exam Room.

5. Which procedures were performed, and why were these needed for the prenatal examination?

 • While still in the Exam Room with Ms. Parlet, click on **Take History**.

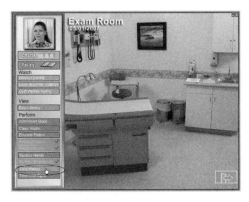

Click on Take History.

- Click on the **Ask** button to view Louise Parlet's answers to the questions regarding her medical history. Document your findings as directed in the program.
- Click **Next** to view additional questions and responses related to the patient's history.
- Complete your documentation. (*Note:* You can return to the previous page to review Ms. Parlet's answers without losing your work.)

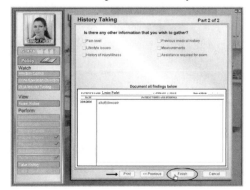

- Click on **Print** to get a hard copy of your documentation, which can be turned in to your instructor.
- Click **Finish** to return to the Exam Room.

Click Print for a hard copy.
Click Finish to return to the Exam Room.

6. What information is important to obtain before a prenatal examination?

7. What information did Louise Parlet provide that might indicate that she is pregnant?

8. How many times has Ms. Parlet conceived? Is she has been pregnant before, what was the outcome?

- Click the exit arrow to get to the **Summary Menu**.
- Click on **Look at Your Performance Summary**. Scroll through the sections to view each wizard you completed and compare your answers with the experts. The summary can also be printed or saved for your instructor.

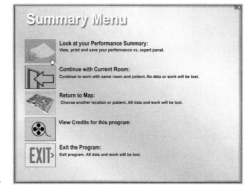

Click on Look at Your Performance Summary.

- Click on **Close** to return to the Summary Menu.
- Click on **Return to Map** and continue to the next exercise.

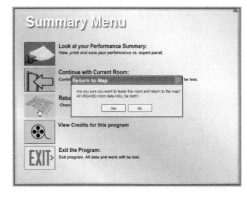

Click on Return to Map.

Exercise 2

 CD-ROM Activity—Assisting with a Gynecologic Examination

 30 minutes

- From the patient list, select **Renee Anderson**. (*Note:* If you have exited the program, sign in again to Mountain View Clinic and select Renee Anderson from the patient list.)

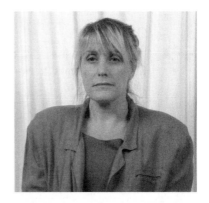

Renee Anderson

- On the office map, highlight **Reception** and click to enter the Reception area.

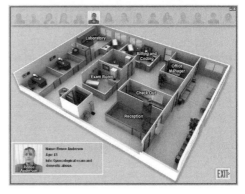

Click on Recpetion.

- Click on **Patient Check-In** to watch the video.
- Click **Close** to return to the Reception desk.

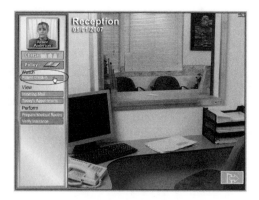

1. What nonverbal communication is most important in this video for the medical assistant to observe and respond to?

2. Did the medical assistant at check-in handle the confidentiality question correctly and accurately? Explain your answer.

➡ • At the Reception desk, click on **Prepare Medical Record** to assemble a chart for Ms. Anderson.

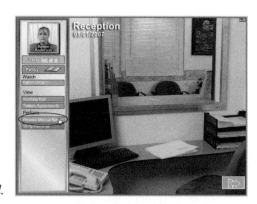

Click on Prepare Medical Record.

- Select **Perform: Assemble Medical Record** to select the forms necessary for Ms. Anderson's visit. The Patient Information tab will automatically open in the bottom portion of the screen.

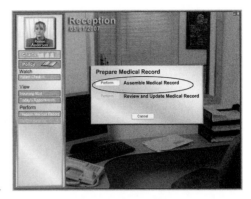

Click on Perform: Assemble Medical Record.

- Under Forms Available, click to select a form that you think should be filed under the Patient Information tab. Click **Add** to confirm the choice. Continue these steps until you are satisfied that you have added all the necessary forms to the Patient Information tab.

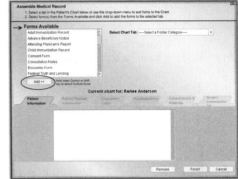

Select and add forms to the Patient Information tab.

- When this tab is complete, move to another tab that you think is necessary for this medical record. To choose a new tab, you can click directly on the chart tab or select from the drop-down menu by clicking the down arrow next to **Select Chart Tab**. Either method will open the selected tab on the bottom half of the screen.

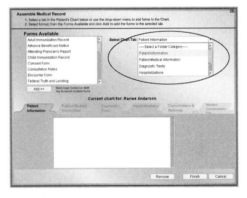

Click on chart tab or choose from the drop-down menu.

- If you wish to remove a chosen form, select the form and click the **Remove** button.

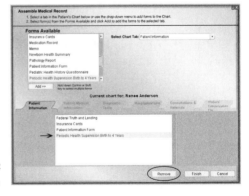

Click Remove to delete a form from the medical record.

- After selecting and filing all the necessary forms under the correct tabs, click **Finish** to close the chart.

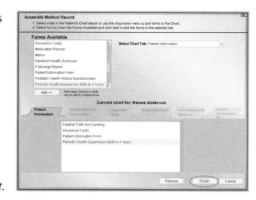

Click Finish to close the chart.

- Click on the exit arrow to leave the Reception area
- From the Summary Menu, select **Look at Your Performance Summary** to compare your answers with the experts. If you missed any answers, consider why those answers you missed were correct.

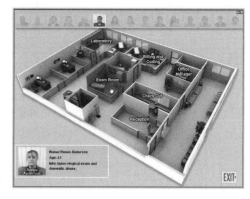

Click on Look at Your Performance Summary.

- Click **Close** to return to the Summary Menu.
- Click **Return to Map** to continue with this exercise.
- Keeping Renee Anderson as your patient, click on **Exam Room** on the office map.

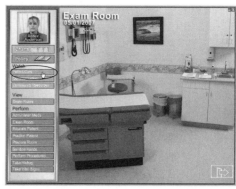

Click on Exam Room.

- Under the Watch heading, click **Patient Care** to view the video.
- At the end of the video, click **Close** to return to the Exam Room.

Click on Patient Care.

3. Susan states that she missed a question on the lab request form concerning previously abnormal Pap smears. Why is this important?

4. During the examination, what nonverbal communication was provided to the medical assistant and physician that might have led to an examination for spousal abuse by the physician?

5. Do you feel that Susan provided the proper verbal and nonverbal support for this patient who had demonstrated distinct nonverbal communication of an emotional problem at check-in? Explain.

6. Why is it important to include the instructions for breast self-examination for each gynecologic patient?

7. Dr. Hayler suggests that Ms. Anderson should have a mammogram. Other than finding a breast lump, what reason would be appropriate for suggesting a mammogram? (*Hint:* Check the chart for the patient's age and health history.)

8. What other information on Ms. Anderson's health history form provides a hint of spousal abuse?

9. When Ms. Anderson arrived for her appointment, medical information was discussed in an ethical and confidential manner. What did Dr. Hayler do later during Ms. Anderson's visit that provides additional evidence of his attempts to maintain guidelines of ethics and confidentiality?

• In the Exam Room, click on **Communication** under the Watch heading to view the video.

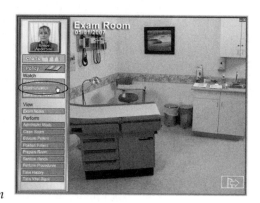

Click on Communication

10. How do you feel about the manner Dr. Hayler used when talking with Ms. Anderson? What about the response of the medical assistant, Susan, to the patient's nonverbal communication?

11. What responsibilities did the medical assistant have concerning the cleaning of the room before Dr. Hayler returned to discuss treatment with Ms. Anderson?

12. True or False:

    _____ The date of the last menstrual period is not important on the lab request for a Pap smear.

    _____ The medical assistant has the distinct responsibility for asking the site of specimen collection during a Pap smear if this information is not provided by the physician.

    _____ When assisting with a pelvic examination, the medical assistant should be near the supply tray to pass needed supplies to the physician but should also be at the patient's side to provide support and observe nonverbal communication.

    _____ With a female patient and a male examiner, the medical assistant has a legal and ethical responsibility to remain in the room at all times.

13. Why is it important that a Pap smear not be collected during the menstrual period and for several days following?

The Pediatric Examination

◯ᴎ **Reading Assignment:** Chapter 24—The Pediatric Examination

Patient: Jade Wong

Objectives:

- Describe the steps necessary in preparing a child for a pediatric examination.
- Explain the differences between obtaining mensurations in children and in adults.
- Plot height and weight on a growth chart for children.
- Describe the role of the medical assistant in a pediatric examination.
- Discuss the importance of effective verbal and nonverbal communication with persons of different cultures.
- Demonstrate the correct documentation of chief complaint with young children.

Exercise 1

 CD-ROM Activity—Assisting with a Pediatric Examination

 45 minutes

- Sign in to Mountain View Clinic.
- From the patient list, select **Jade Wong**.

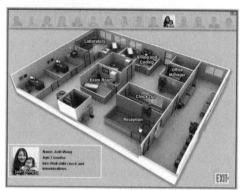

Jade Wong

- On the office map, highlight and click on **Reception** to enter the Reception area.

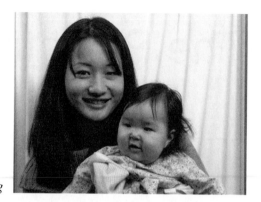

Click on Reception.

- Under the Perform heading, click on **Prepare Medical Record**.

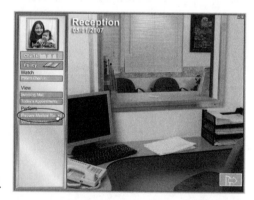

Click on Prepare Medical Record.

- Select **Perform: Assemble Medical Record** to select the forms necessary for Jade's visit. The Patient Information tab will open automatically.

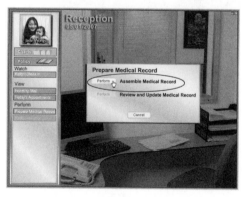

Click on Assemble Medical Record.

➤ • From the Forms Available list, choose the forms that should be filed under the Patient Information tab. Click **Add** to confirm your choice.

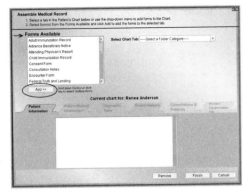

Select and add forms to the Patient Information tab.

• When the Patient Information tab is complete, move to each of the other tabs that you think are necessary to prepare this patient's medical record. To select a new tab, you may either click on the tab on the medical record or use the drop-down menu next to Select Chart Tab. Continue selecting forms to fill the tabs in Jade Wong's medical record.

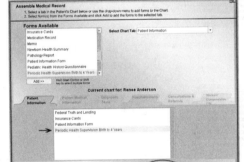

Select new tabs by clicking on the tabs or by using the drop-down menu.

• If you wish to remove a chosen form, highlight the form and click the **Remove** button.

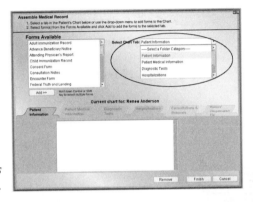

Click Remove to delete a form from the medical record.

• After selecting and filing all the necessary forms under the correct tabs, click **Finish** to close the chart.

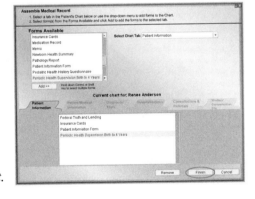

Click Finish to close the chart.

- Click on the exit arrow at the bottom of screen to leave the Reception area. From the Summary Menu, select **Look at Your Performance Summary** to compare your answers with those of the experts. How did you do?

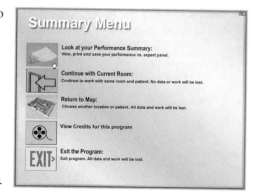

Click on Look at Your Performance Summary.

- Click **Close** to return to the Summary Menu.
- Click **Return to Map** to continue with this exercise. Keeping Jade Wong as the patient, click on **Exam Room** on the office map.

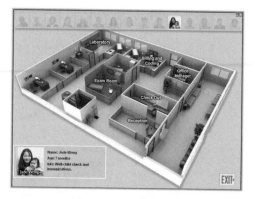

Click on Exam Room.

- Under the Watch heading, select **Well-Baby Visit** and watch the video.
- Click **Close** at the end of the video to return to the Exam Room.

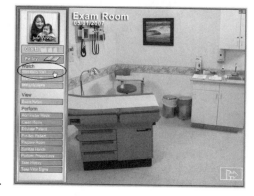

Click on Well-Baby Visit.

1. What measurements would you expect the medical assistant to obtain for Jade's well-baby visit?

2. Why is it important for the medical assistant to develop rapport with a child and with parents when assisting with a well-child office visit?

3. As the medical assistant works with Jade, she is using the father as an interpreter and is allowing the mother to have an active part in the medical care through this means. Do you feel this is an important part of the care, or do you believe the medical assistant should provide care and speak only with the father? Explain your answer.

4. In what way is the preparation of a child for a pediatric examination similar to the preparation of an adult for an examination?

5. Why is it important to remove an infant's clothing before weighing? Why should the diaper be removed?

6. What are some of the differences between the preparation of a child for an examination versus the preparation of an adult for an examination?

7. What tactics may be used with older children to gain their confidence?

8. What roles do verbal and nonverbal communication play in a pediatric examination?

→ • Remain in the Exam Room with Jade and select **Position Patient** under the Perform heading.

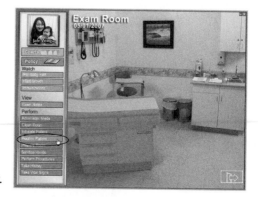

Click on Position Patient.

• Select all positions Jade will be placed in during her exam.
• Click **Finish** to return to the Exam Room.
• Click the exit arrow to go to the Summary Menu.
• On the Summary Menu, click on **Look at Your Performance Summary**.

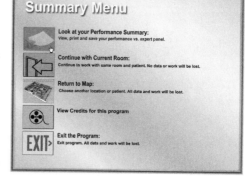

Click on Look at Your Performance Summary.

• Scroll down to the relevant section and compare your answers with those of the experts. The summary can be printed or saved for your instructor.
• Click **Close** to return to the Summary Menu.
• Click on **Return to Map** to continue the lesson.

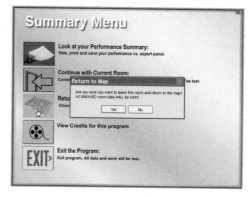

Click on Return to Map.

➙ • Continue with Jade Wong as the patient. On the office map, highlight and click on **Billing and Coding**.

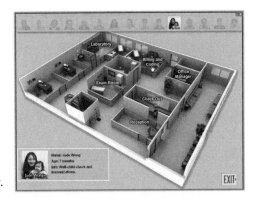

Click on Billing and Coding.

• Open Jade's chart by clicking on **Charts**.

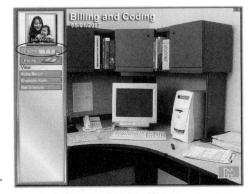

Click on Charts.

• Click on the **Patient Medical Information** tab and select **6-Newborn Health Summary** to review some of Jade's past medical history.

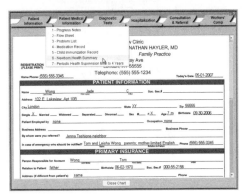

Select 6-Newborn Health Summary.

• Determine Jade's birth weight and length from the medical history in the Newborn Health Summary.

9. On the growth chart below, plot Jade's birth weight and length as recorded in the Newborn Health Summary. Document your findings in the box in the lower right corner of the chart, including the measurement for head cirumference. In the Comment section, note Jade's weight and length as they compare with national percentiles.

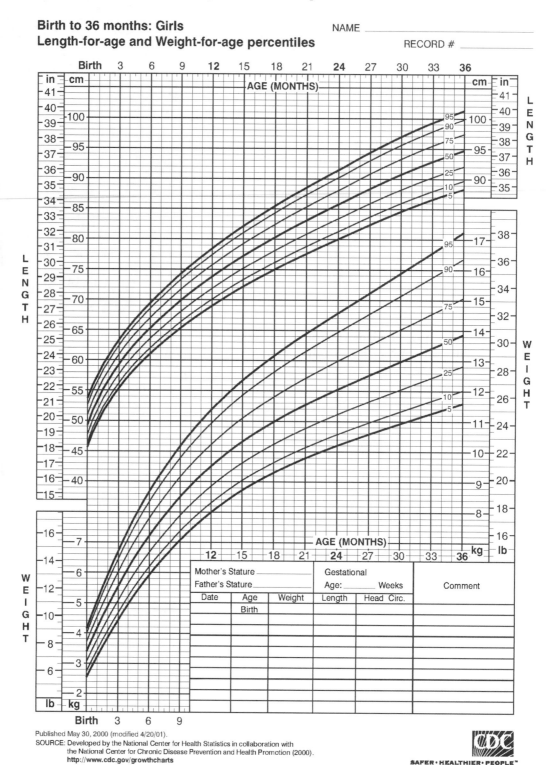

Birth to 36 months: Girls
Length-for-age and Weight-for-age percentiles

NAME _____

RECORD # _____

Published May 30, 2000 (modified 4/20/01).
SOURCE: Developed by the National Center for Health Statistics in collaboration with
the National Center for Chronic Disease Prevention and Health Promotion (2000).
http://www.cdc.gov/growthcharts

• Click again on the **Patient Medical Information** tab and select **1-Progress Notes**.

- Determine Jade's weight, length, head circumference, and chest circumference recorded from today's visit.

10. On the same growth chart used in question 9, plot Jade's measurements from today's visit. Document your new findings in the box in the lower right corner of the chart and note the new percentiles for Jade in the Comment section.

11. What was Jade's percentile of weight at birth? What was her percentile of length at birth?

12. Does Mr. Wong's observation that Jade looks small have any foundation, according to the growth chart for her findings today? Explain your answer.

 • Look again at the Progress Notes and read the chief complaint documented for today's visit.

13. Why is the chief complaint in quotation marks?

14. True or False:

a. _____ The growth charts are the same for both gender and for all ages.

b. _____ A well-baby visit is usually scheduled every 2 months for the first 6 months so that the child can receive the needed immunizations on schedule.

c. _____ After the age 6 months, the well-baby visits are scheduled every 3 months until age 18 months.

d. _____ After 2 years of age, well-child visits are scheduled every 2 years.

e. _____ The medical assistant should obtain information about the motor and cognitive development of the child at each visit.

f. _____ If a child is seen for a sick child visit between well-baby visits, the child does not need to have weight and length obtained.

g. _____ When measuring the circumference of the head and chest, the measurement should be taken at the greatest circumference.

h. _____ Infant scales measure weight in pounds and ounces rather than in pounds and fractions of pounds as with adult scales.

i. _____ When measuring the height of an infant, the measurement should be from the heel to the crown of the head.

j. _____ When a child is able to stand, the child may be weighed on balance beam scales with no difficulty.

k. _____ When weighing a young child who is afraid of the balance beam scales or who weighs more than the infant scale can accommodate, an alternative is to weigh the mother and child together on an adult scale and then weigh the mother alone. After obtaining the two weights, you can determine the weight of the child by subtracting the mother's weight from the combined weight of the two.

Assisting with Minor Office Surgery

Reading Assignment: Chapter 25—Minor Office Surgery

Patients: Jose Imero, Tristan Tsosie

Objectives:

- Describe the instruments and supplies needed for suturing of simple lacerations and for removal of sutures.
- Discuss the correct procedure for preparing the patient for suturing of a laceration.
- Distinguish between supplies that should be sterile and those that can simply be aseptically clean for the removal of sutures.
- Describe the importance of infection control and sterile aseptic technique with minor surgery.
- Describe the need for correct dispensing of biohazardous materials when performing wound care.
- Discuss the need for patient education following suturing of a laceration and suture removal.

Exercise 1

 CD-ROM Activity—Assisting with Minor Office Surgery

 45 minutes

- Sign in to Mountain View Clinic.
- From the patient list, select **Jose Imero**.

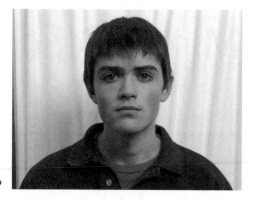

Jose Imero

- On the office map, highlight and click on **Exam Room**.

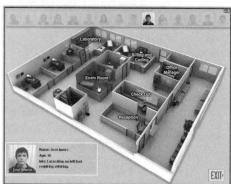

Click on Exam Room.

- Click on **Exam Notes** to read the documentation regarding Jose's visit. Note the procedures he is to have performed during his exam. Click **Finish** to return to the Exam Room.
- Under the Perform heading, select **Prepare Room** to select the supplies needed for Jose's visit. (*Note:* You can reopen the Exam Notes for reference as you make your selections.)

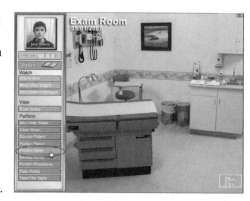

Click on Prepare Room.

- Select the first item needed for Jose's visit from the alphabetical list and click **Add Item** to confirm your choice. The items you select will appear in the Selected Supplies column.
- Repeat this step until you are satisfied you have everything you need from the list.

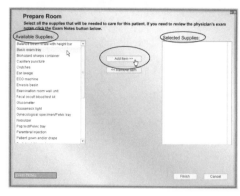

Select the supplies needed for this visit.

- Do NOT close this window. Keep the Prepare Room wizard open as you continue with the lesson.

- In the Prepare Room wizard, click on **Wound Care** in the list of Available Supplies and review the contents on the tray shown in the photo.

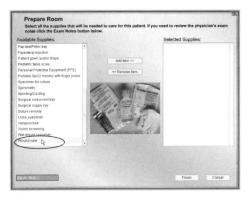

Select Wound Care from the list of Available Supplies.

1. Below, list the supplies (in any order) provided for wound care as shown in the Prepare Room wizard photo. Also briefly explain why each is needed.

Supplied Item   **Reason for Use**
_____

- Still in the Prepare Room wizard, select **Surgical Supply Tray** from the list of Available Supplies and review the tray's contents as shown in the photo.

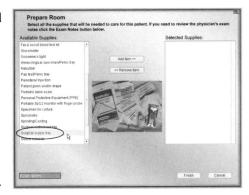

Click on Surgical Supply Tray.

2. What disposable supplies are found on the supply tray that will be needed for the suturing of Jose's foot? (*Note:* You can check your answers when you watch the video later in this exercise.)

→ • Next, click on **Surgical Instrument Tray** in the Available Supplies list. Again, review the tray's contents as shown in the photo.

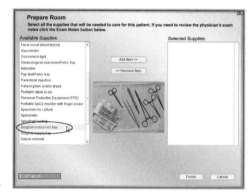

Click on Surgical Instrument Tray.

3. What instruments and supplies are found on the tray that could possibly be used for suturing Jose's foot?

4. Dr. Hayler specifically states that he is going to probe Jose's wound for possible foreign objects. With that information, what sterile materials necessary for preparing to suture a laceration are missing from the surgical instrument tray?

5. Match each of the following surgical instruments with its use or description.

Instrument	**Use or Description**
_____ Scalpel	a. Used to find foreign objects in a wound
_____ Forceps	b. Used for grasping and squeezing
_____ Operating scissors	c. Used to open orifices
_____ Hemostats	d. Have straight sharp blades for cutting through tissue
_____ Needle holders	e. Small surgical knife used to cut through tissue
_____ Retractors	f. Used to pull back tissue and skin
_____ Speculum	g. Forceps-like instrument used to hold circular needles
_____ Suture scissors	h. Used to clamp blood vessels and to hold tissue
_____ Probe	i. Forceps with straight sharp points for removing foreign objects from wounds
_____ Splinter forceps	j. Scissors used to cut sutures

 • Click **Finish** to close the Prepare Room wizard and return to the Exam Room.

• Under the Watch heading, click on **Wound Care** to view the video.

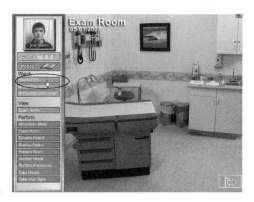

Click on Wound Care.

• At the end of the video, click **Close** to return to the Exam Room (*Remember:* You can click on the play button if you wish to replay the video.)

6. Why is the red bag on the Mayo stand?

7. Why did Charlie place a protective sheet under Jose's leg?

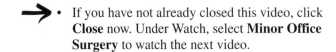 • If you have not already closed this video, click **Close** now. Under Watch, select **Minor Office Surgery** to watch the next video.

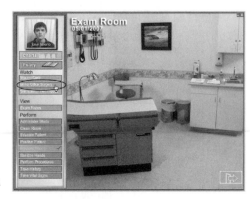

Click on Minor Office Surgery.

• While watching this video, look for a distinct break in sterile technique.

8. What is the break in sterile technique that Charlie allows to happen?

9. Why was it important that Charlie pass the suture material around the surgical tray?

10. True or False:

   a. _____ The medical assistant is responsible for supplying a light source when assisting with minor surgery.

   b. _____ When setting a sterile field, the entire area is considered sterile.

   c. _____ When preparing a tray for suturing during minor surgery, time efficiency would best be served by placing the instruments in the order of use.

   d. _____ All surgical trays must be prepared by the medical assistant according to the desires of the physician.

e. _____ Once a minor surgery suture tray has been set, the medical assistant cannot add instruments or supplies to the tray.

f. _____ Surgical scissors may have sharp blades, blunt blades, or a combination of the two.

g. _____ When assisting with minor surgery, the medical assistant must always use sterile gloves.

h. _____ The application of sterile gloves requires a different technique than that of the application of nonsterile gloves.

i. _____ When pouring a solution onto a sterile field, the medical assistant should first pour and discard the solution over the lip of the container and then pour onto the sterile field.

j. _____ When opening a sterile pack, the flap toward you should be opened first.

k. _____ Suture material is always the same for each wound and each physician.

l. _____ Suture material comes in absorbable and nonabsorbable types.

m. _____ Absorbable suture is usually used for subcutaneous tissue and below the outer skin.

n. _____ Nonabsorbable suture is usually used for deep tissue.

o. _____ Suture material comes in varying sizes, lengths, and absorbability.

p. _____ Skin may be closed with staples and adhesive skin closures.

q. _____ Selection of suture material depends on the site, length, and depth of the wound.

• Click **Close** and the exit arrow to leave the Exam Room.
• Click **Return to Map**.

Exercise 2

 CD-ROM Activity—Assisting with Suture Removal

 20 minutes

• From the patient list, select **Tristan Tsosie**. (*Note:* If you have exited the program, sign in again to Mountain View Clinic and select Tristan Tsosie from the patient list.)

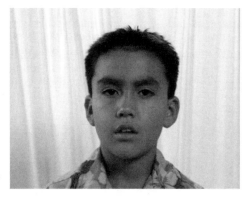

Tristan Tsosie

• On the office map, highlight and click on **Exam Room**.

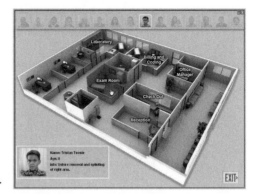

Click on Exam Room.

• Under Perform, click on **Prepare Room** to select the supplies needed for Tristan's visit.

• From the list of Available Supplies, select **Suture Removal** and review the tray's contents as shown in the photo.

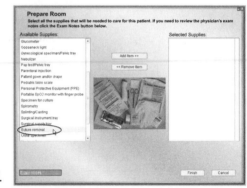

Click on Suture Removal.

1. List the items shown on the tray.

2. Since the sutures are to be removed after a wound culture has been obtained, when should the cleansing of the wound take place?

3. The medical assistant is preparing Tristan for the removal of sutures. Tristan asks whether the procedure is going to hurt. Should the medical assistant answer the question before continuing with the procedure, or is it effective verbal communication to ignore the question?

4. When removing sutures, what supplies should be sterile and what supplies can be aseptically clean?

5. True or False:

   a. _____ Before removing sutures, the medical assistant should obtain the permission of the physician.

   b. _____ If the wound appears to gape open during suture removal and the physician has stated the all sutures should be removed, the medical assistant should continue to remove the sutures.

   c. _____ When sutures are being removed, the patient should be placed in a comfortable position to prevent injury or unnecessary discomfort.

   d. _____ All sutures will be ready to be removed at the same time following injury.

   e. _____ The size and location of the wound are important factors in deciding when sutures will be removed.

   f. _____ All sutures may be removed using the same size of suture scissors and forceps.

   g. _____ When sutures are being removed, the suture should be cut as close to the skin as possible and then pulled in the opposite direction to prevent the microorganisms from passing through the skin into the wound.

   h. _____ When cleansing the area before removing sutures, the skin should be thoroughly cleansed and the exudate removed.

   i. _____ When removing sutures, it is not important to count the sutures removed, since you only need to remove those you can see.

• Returning to the Prepare Room wizard, select the first item needed for Tristan's visit from the alphabetical list and click **Add Item** to confirm your choice. The items you select will appear in the Selected Supplies column.

• Repeat this step until you are satisfied you have everything you need from the list. (*Note:* The Exam Notes are available if you need to refer to them.)

• Click **Finish** to return to the Exam Room.

• In the Exam Room, select **Clean Room** (under Perform) and select the necessary steps to be taken at the end of Tristan's visit.

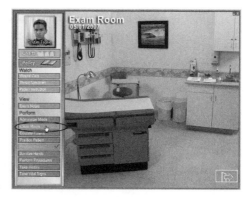

Click on Clean Room.

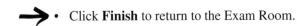 • Click **Finish** to return to the Exam Room.

6. Explain the importance of proper care of the wound at home after suturing and suture removal.

7. Below, document the removal of sutures from a clean wound on Tristan Tsosie's leg. The sutures were inserted 6 days earlier. Be sure to document that the physician, Dr. Hayler, has observed the sutures and has told you to remove these 10 sutures. Also document the dressing of the wound following removal and indicate that the patient did not seem to have any problems. Use today's date for the documentation and your initials for the entry.

DATE	PATIENT VISITS AND FINDINGS

PATIENT'S NAME _____ ☐ FEMALE ☐ MALE   Date of Birth: __/__/__

ALLERGIC TO _____

PAGE ____ of ____

ORDER #25-7133-01 • ©1999 BIBBERO SYSTEMS, INC. • PETALUMA, CA   TO REORDER CALL 800-BIBBERO (800-242-2376) OR FAX (800) 242-9330 MFD IN USA

• Click the exit arrow to get to the Summary Menu.
• Select **Look at Your Performance Summary** to compare your answers for Tristan Tsosie with those of the experts.
• Select **Return to Map** to move on to the next lesson or select **Exit** to close the program.

Administration of Medication and Intravenous Therapy

/OⱭ **Reading Assignment:** Chapter 26—Administration of Medication and
Intravenous Therapy

Patients: Shaunti Begay, Jesus Santo, Jade Wong

Objectives:

- Describe preparation of medications according to physician's orders.
- Discuss the steps necessary to administer a parenteral injection according to physician's orders.
- Describe the preparation of a patient for the administration of medication.
- Identify the necessary steps for patient safety with the administration of medications.
- Identify local resources for immunizations and for patient education.

Exercise 1

  CD-ROM Activity—Administering Parenteral Medications

20 minutes

- Sign in to Mountain View Clinic.
- From the patient list, select **Jesus Santo**.

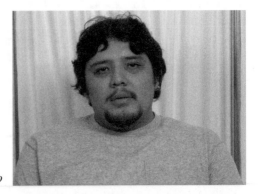

Jesus Santo

- On the office map, highlight and click on **Exam Room**.

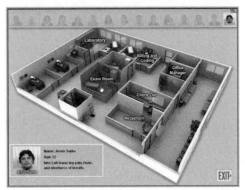

Click on Exam Room.

- Click on **Exam Notes** (under View) and read the documentation on Mr. Santo's visit for today.

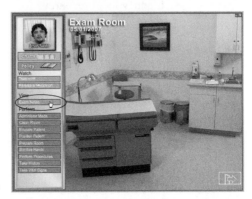

Click on Exam Notes.

- Click **Finish** to return to the Exam Room.
- Under the Perform heading, click on **Prepare Room** to select the supplies needed for Mr. Santo's visit. (*Note:* You can reopen the Exam Notes for reference as you make your selections.)

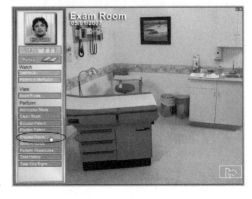

Click on Prepare Room.

- Select the first item needed for Mr. Santo's visit from the alphabetical list and click **Add Item** to confirm your choice. The items you select will appear in the Selected Supplies column.

- Repeat this step until you are satisfied you have everything you need from the list.

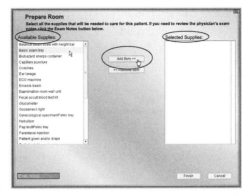

Select the supplies needed for this visit.

- Do NOT close this window. Keep the Prepare Room wizard open as you continue with the lesson.

1. The medical assistant is asked to prepare Bicillin-LA 1,200,000 units for injection. If the medication is available as Bicillin-LA 600,000 units/mL, how many milliliters would Charlie prepare to give Mr. Santo?

2. Why is the classification of the Bicillin-LA?

- In the Prepare Room wizard, click on **Parenteral Injection** in the list of Available Supplies and review the contents on the tray shown in the photo.

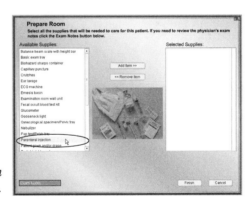

Select Parenteral Injection from the list of Available Supplies.

3. On the parenteral injection tray are four syringes, a tuberculin syringe, a 5-mL syringe, an insulin syringe, and a 3-mL syringe. Which is the correct syringe for the administration of the medication ordered?

4. Below, choose the correct syringe and mark it to indicate the amount of medication that should be given to Mr. Santo.

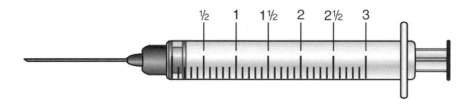

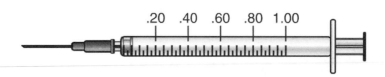

➡ • Click **Finish** to close the Prepare Room wizard and return to the Exam Room.

5. Where should the syringe be disposed following the administration of the Bicillin-LA?
   a. In the regular waste container
   b. In the biohazard waste container
   c. In the puncture-proof biohazard waste container

6. Where should the used supplies, other than the syringe, be disposed following the administration of Bicillin-LA?
   a. In the regular waste container
   b. In the biohazard waste container
   c. In the puncture-proof biohazard waste container

7. Below, properly document the injection given to Mr. Santo, using the present date and time.

8. The Exam Notes state that the CBC should be drawn prior to administration of the Bicillin LA. Why should the CBC be drawn first and then the medication administered?

9. Why is it important for Mr. Santo to stay in the office for 15 to 20 minutes following the injection of Bicillin LA?

10. The physician has stated in the Exam Notes that the patient should wait for 15 to 20 minutes before leaving the office. Mr. Santo was brought to the medical office by his employer, Mr. Freeman. If Mr. Freeman does not want to wait, what should the medical assistant at the check-out desk do?

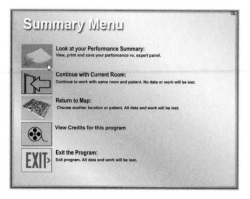

- • Click the exit arrow to get to the Summary Menu.
- • Select **Look at Your Performance Summary** to compare your answers for Jesus Santo with those of the experts.

Click on Look at Your Performance Summary.

- • Select **Return to Map** to move on to the next exercise.

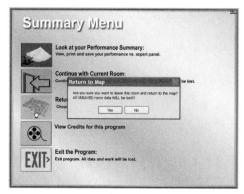

Click on Return to Map.

Exercise 2

 CD-ROM Activity—Administering and Documenting Immunizations

 30 minutes

- • From the patient list, select **Shaunti Begay**. (*Note:* If you have exited the program, sign in again to Mountain View Clinic and select Shaunti Begay from the patient list.)

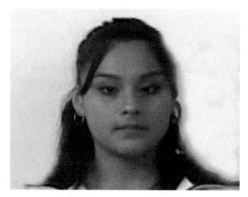

Shaunti Begay

- On the office map, highlight and click on the **Exam Room**.

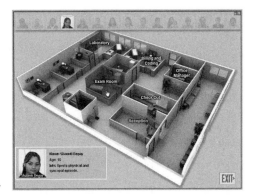

Click on Exam Room.

- Under the Watch heading, select **Immunizations** to view the video.

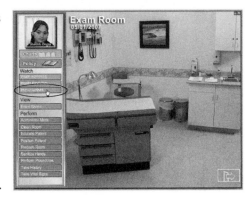

Click on Immunization.

- At the end of the video, click **Close** to return to the Exam Room.

1. What is the site of the hepatitis B immunization?

2. When is the next dose of hepatitis B due?

- Click the exit arrow to get to the Summary Menu.
- On the Summary Menu, click on **Return to Map**.
- On the office map, highlight and click on **Check Out** to review the end of Shaunti's visit.

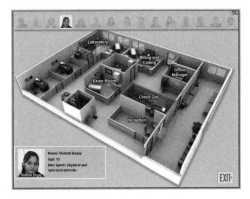

Click on Check Out.

• Click on **Charts** to open Shaunti's medical record.

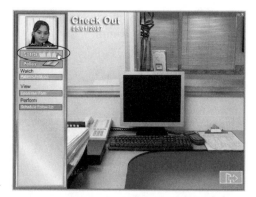

Click on Charts.

• Click on the **Patient Medical Information** tab and select **2-Progress Notes** to view the documentation of Shaunti's exam.

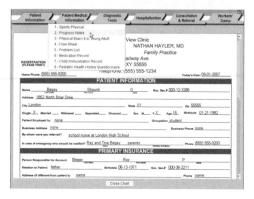

Click on 2-Progress Notes.

• Read the documentation regarding Shaunti's immunization.

3. What volume of hepatitis B vaccine is being given to Shaunti?

4. Below, indicate the amount of vaccine that should be administered to Shaunti for the hepatitis B immunization.

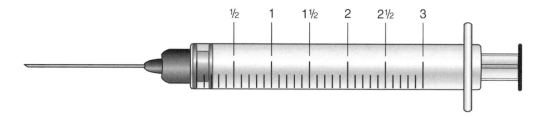

5. What is the expiration date of the hepatitis B vaccine?

6. What is a VIS statement? Why is this required for an immunization?

7. When the hepatitis B vaccine is being prepared for administration, when should the medical assistant check the medication against the physician's order prior to administering?

8. What are the seven rights of medication administration?

9. Why is it important to document the manufacturer of an immunizing agent, as well as the lot number and expiration date?

→ • Click **Close Chart** to return to the Check Out area.
   • Click the exit arrow to get to the Summary Menu.
   • Click on **Return to Map** to continue to the next exercise.

Exercise 3

 CD-ROM Activity—Immunizations as Indicated in Well-Child Visits

 25 minutes

- From the patient list, select **Jade Wong**. (*Note:* If you have exited the program, sign in again to Mountain View Clinic and select Jade Wong from the patient list.)

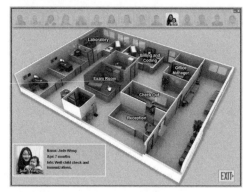

Jade Wong

- On the office map, highlight and click on **Exam Room**.

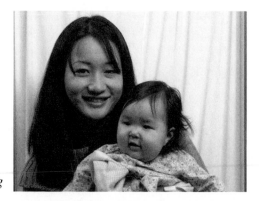

Click on Exam Room.

- Under the Watch heading, select **Immunizations** to view the video.

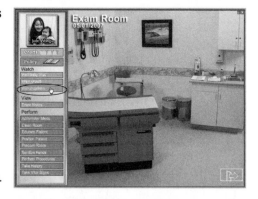

Click on Immunizations.

- At the end of the video, click **Close** to return to the Exam Room.
- Under the View heading, click on **Exam Notes** to read the documentation of Jade's visit.

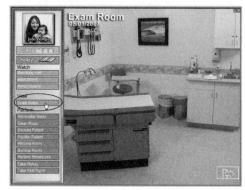

Click on Exam Notes.

1. Why is it important to provide the parents with information, including the VIS, concerning the immunizations that the child will receive?

2. The medical assistant asked whether Jade had any problems with previous immunizations. Why is this information important before administering the immunizations at this visit?

3. What immunizations will be given to Jade? Be sure to include the diseases that these immunizations protect against (not just the abbreviations of the immunizations).

4. The Exam Notes indicate that Jade's mother has not received the polio vaccine. Why is the injectable polio vaccine safer for the mother?

5. What resources are available in your community for the mother to obtain the polio vaccine if she wants to get it some place other than the physician's office?

• Click on **Finish** to return to the Exam Room.
- Click on the exit arrow to get to the Summary Menu.
- On the Summary Menu, click on **Return to Map** to continue the lesson.
- On the office map, click on **Check Out** to review the end of Jade's visit.
- At the Check Out desk, click on **Charts**. Next, click on the **Patient Medical Information** tab and select **1-Progress Notes**.
- Read the final documentation of Jade's exam.

6. In the Progress Notes, the medical assistant states that Jade seemed to tolerate the immunizations with no problems. Why is this documentation important?

7. What volume of Pediarix will be administered to Jade?

8. Indicate on the syringe below the volume of Pediarix that Jade should receive.

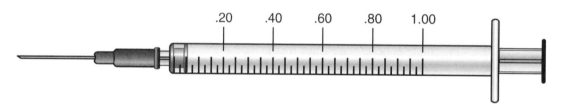

9. Below, document the immunizations that have been given to Jade today. Be sure to follow CDC guidelines.

Vaccine Administration Record
for Children and Teens

Patient name: _____

Birthdate: _____

Chart number: _____

Before administering any vaccines, give the parent/guardian all appropriate copies of Vaccine Information Statements (VISs) and make sure they understand the risks and benefits of the vaccine(s). Update the patient's personal record card or provide a new one whenever you administer vaccine.

Vaccine	Type of Vaccine* (generic abbreviation)	Date given (mo/day/yr)	Route	Site given (RA, LA, RT, LT)	Vaccine		Vaccine Information Statement		Signature/ initials of vaccinator
					lot #	mfr.	Date on VIS§	Date given§	
Hepatitis B† (e.g., HepB, Hib-HepB, DTaP-HepB-IPV)			IM						
			IM						
			IM						
			IM						
Diphtheria, Tetanus, Pertussis† (e.g, DTaP, DT, DTaP-Hib, DTaP-HepB-IPV, Td)			IM						
			IM						
			IM						
			IM						
			IM						
			IM						
Haemophilus influenzae type b† (e.g., Hib, Hib-HepB, DTaP-Hib)			IM						
			IM						
			IM						
			IM						
Polio† (e.g, IPV, DTaP-HepB-IPV)			IM•SC						
			IM•SC						
			IM•SC						
			IM•SC						
Pneumococcal conjugate (PCV)			IM						
			IM						
			IM						
			IM						
Measles, Mumps, Rubella (MMR)			SC						
			SC						
Varicella (Var)			SC						
			SC						
Hepatitis A** (HepA)			IM						
			IM						
Influenza** (Flu)			IM						
			IM						
			IM						
			IM						
			IM						
Other**									
Other**									

*Record the generic abbreviation for the type of vaccine given (e.g., DTaP-Hib, PCV), *not* the trade name.

†For combination vaccines, fill in the row for each individual antigen composing the combination.

§Record the publication date of each VIS as well as the date it is given to the patient. According to federal law, VISs must be given to patients (or parent/guardian of a minor child) before administering each dose of DTaP, Td, Hib, polio, MMR, varicella, PCV, or HepB vaccine, or combinations thereof.

**Influenza, pneumococcal polysaccharide (PPV23), hepatitis A, and/or meningococcal vaccines are recommended for certain high-risk children.

www.immunize.org/catg.d/p2022b.pdf • Item #P2022 (4/03)

Immunization Action Coalition • 1573 Selby Avenue • St. Paul, MN 55104 • (651) 647-9009 • www.immunize.org

10. Why is the use of a 1-mL syringe more appropriate when administering the medication to Jade?

→ • Click **Close Chart** to return to the Check Out desk.

• Under the Watch heading, select **Patient Check-Out** to view the video.

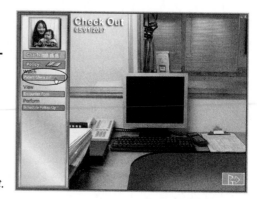

Click on Patient Check-Out.

11. The medical assistant provides Jade's father, Mr. Wong, with information concerning child nutrition and community resources. She indicates that Mr. Wong and his wife are open to this help. Why is it important that the implied permission is provided, either verbally or nonverbally, prior to giving information?

12. The Progress Notes also state that Jade's mother has been referred to ESL classes. What does ESL mean?

13. Using the Internet or a local resource guide, list the local resources for ESL education.

Cardiopulmonary Procedures: Electrocardiogram

∞ Reading Assignment: Chapter 27—Cardiopulmonary Procedures

Patient: John R. Simmons

Objectives:

- Discuss the purpose of electrocardiography (ECG).
- Discuss the correct placement of leads for ECG.
- Explain the electrical conduction system of the heart.
- Identify the components of the cardiac cycle.
- State the need for quality control and the use of standardization marks.
- Discuss the proper handling of ECG paper and the means of tracing the cardiac cycle.
- Describe patient preparation for an ECG.
- Identify the 12 leads found on an electrocardiogram.
- Explain artifacts and the causes.
- Discuss professionalism and ethical behavior when performing electrocardiography.

Exercise 1

 Writing Activity—Understanding the Purpose and Components of an Electrocardiogram

 45 minutes

1. What is electrocardiography?

2. Describe the electrical conduction of the heart from the inception at the SA node through the electrical impulses to the fibers of the ventricles.

3. Label the diagram below to show the anatomy of the heart.

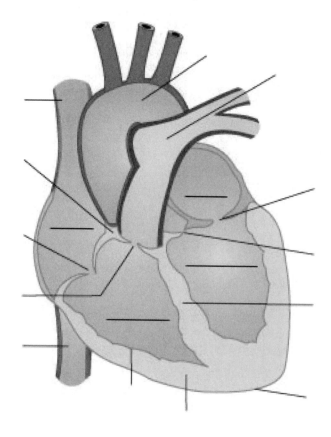

4. On the diagram below, label the components of the electrical conduction system.

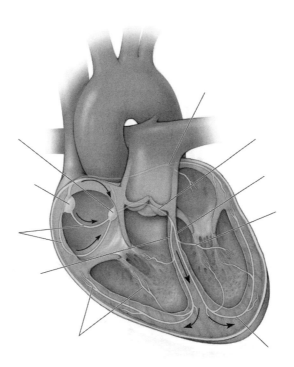

5. Using the diagrams in questions 3 and 4 for reference, match the columns below to show the movement of blood through the heart and lungs. (*Hint:* Begin at the superior/inferior vena cava, which returns deoxygenated blood to the heart.)

Order of Movement in Heart   **Region of the Heart**

_____ 1st area   a. Superior/inferior vena cava

_____ 2nd area   b. Right atria

_____ 3rd area   c. Tricuspid valve

_____ 4th area   d. Right ventricle

_____ 5th area   e. Pulmonary semilunar valve

_____ 6th area   f. Pulmonary arteries

_____ 7th area   g. Lungs

_____ 8th area   h. Pulmonary veins

_____ 9th area   i. Left atria

_____ 10th area   j. Bicuspid valve

_____ 11th area   k. Left ventricles

_____ 12th area   l. Aortic semilunar valves

_____ 13th area   m. Aorta

6. Label the the waves, segments, and intervals on the ECG tracing below.

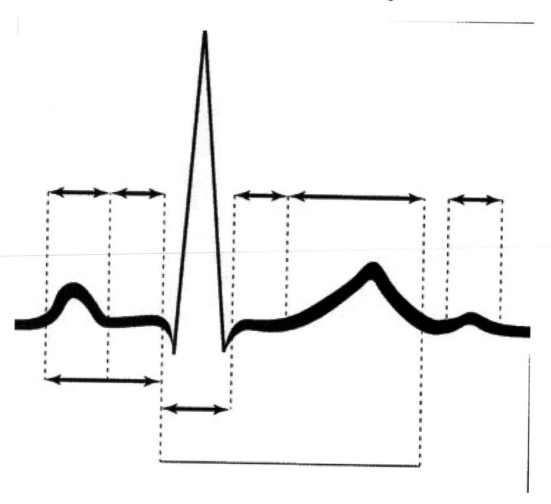

7. What does a wave on an electrocardiogram tracing indicate?

8. What does a segment on an electrocardiogram tracing indicate?

9. What does an interval on an electrocardiogram tracing indicate?

10. What does the QRS complex indicate on an electrocardiogram tracing?

11. How does the physician use electrocardiograph paper to interpret the tracing?

12. Why is it important that the ECG tracing be handled carefully and not be allowed to smear or be folded in any way?

13. What is the purpose of the standardization mark on an electrocardiogram? How is it used?

14. a. When the electrical impulse arrives and the heart muscle is ready to contract, this is called _____.

    b. When the electrical impulse is received and the heart muscle contracts, this is called

    _____.

    c. When the electrical impulse ends and the heart muscle is at rest, this is called

    _____.

15. What electrical activity of the heart is indicated by the P wave?

16. What electrical activity is indicated by the T wave?

Exercise 2

CD-ROM Activity—Preparing for the Electrocardiogram

30 minutes

1. On the diagram below, show the locations and the markings of the leads to be placed for obtaining an electrocardiograph.

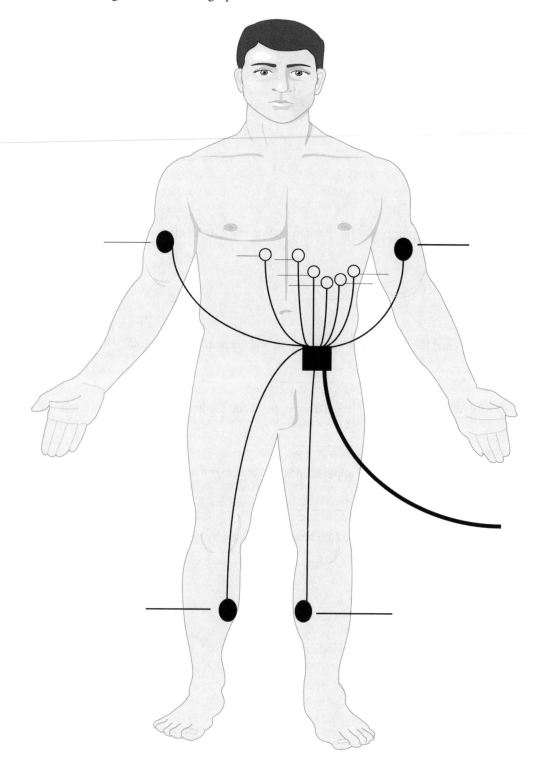

2. If Dr. Simmons had a limb amputation or a bandage or cast on one of his extremities, how would the ECG lead be placed?

3. How should electrodes be placed on patients who have lesions, wounds, or incisions on the chest?

4. Mrs. Glassman is to have an ECG. She is obese and has pendulous breasts. How can you place the electrodes on this patient?

5. What clothing should Mrs. Glassman remove for accurate placement of the electrodes?

6. Which electrode placed on the body is the ground wire for the ECG?

7. What do the bipolar leads trace? Which leads of the electrocardiogram are the bipolar leads?

8. What does a rhythm strip show on the ECG? Which lead provides this information?

• Sign in to Mountain View Clinic.
  • From the patient list, select **John R. Simmons**.

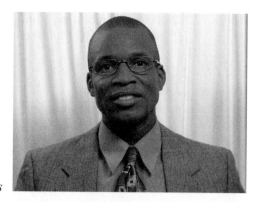

John R. Simmons

  • On the office map, highlight and click on **Exam Room** to enter the examination area.

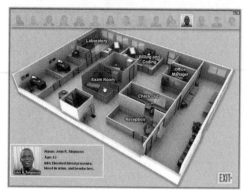

Click on Exam Room.

  • Under the Watch heading, select **ECG Testing** to begin viewing the video. Pause the video at the first fade-out by clicking the control button on the far left.

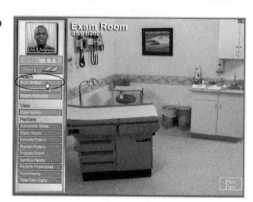

Click on ECG Testing.

9. Describe Dr. Simmons' position on the table and how he is dressed. Do you think that he has been appropriately prepared for the ECG?

10. Is it always necessary to remove the patient's shoes and socks when performing an ECG? Why or why not?

11. Dr. Simmons asked Danielle, the medical assisting extern, whether everything was all right. He also stated that his hand was itching during the ECG. Why do you think Dr. Simmons tried to offer a reason for there being a problem with ECG?

12. Imagine that you were the patient. What reaction do you think you would have if you saw such a perplexed look on the medical assisting extern's face?

13. Danielle then stated that the recording was "fuzzy." What are fuzzy lines on the electrocardiograph called? What causes these lines?

14. What steps did Danielle take to correct this problem? What other steps could have been taken if her initial attempts had not corrected the problem?

15. Why is it important for Danielle to be sure the abnormal tracing is an artifact rather than a dysrhythmia?

• Let's return to the video. Click the play button to continue watching. As you observe the video, consider whether you think Danielle acts professionally.

• Once again, pause the video at the next fade-out.

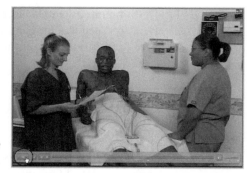

Click the pause button to temporarily stop the video.

16. Do you think Danielle acted in a professional manner when discussing the ECG tracing with Dr. Simmons? Explain your answer.

 • Click the play button and watch the remainder of the video.

17. Do you feel that the medical assistant correctly handled the fact that Danielle had discussed the ECG tracing with Dr. Simmons? Explain your answer.

18. On the blank Progress Notes below, document the obtaining of the electrocardiograph on Dr. Simmons. Use today's date and time for the documentation.

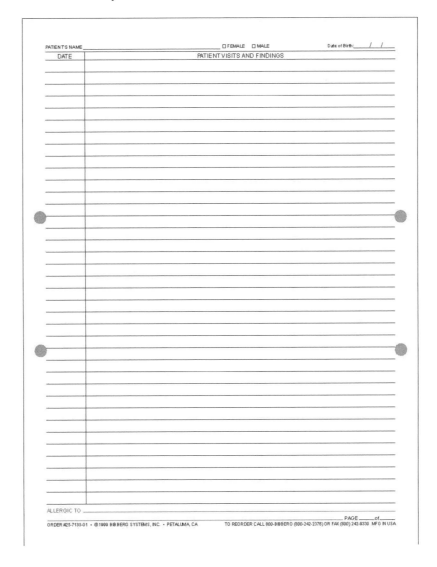

Cardiopulmonary Procedures: Pulmonary Function Testing

Reading Assignment: Chapter 27—Cardiopulmonary Procedures

Patients: John R. Simmons, Hu Huang

Objectives:

- Describe certain respiratory functioning tests.
- Discuss how oxygen and carbon dioxide levels may be measured.
- List indications for pulmonary function testing.
- Describe the meaning of FVC, FEV_1, and FEV_1/FVC ratio.
- List the necessary steps in patient preparation for respiratory testing.
- Explain the calibration of a spirometer.
- Describe the role of the medical assistant in spirometry testing.
- Describe the role of the medical assistant in collection of a sputum specimen.

Exercise 1

Writing Activity—Elements in Respiratory Testing

15 minutes

1. What are the purposes of pulmonary function tests?

2. How does spirometry testing provide information concerning the condition of the lungs?

3. List at least three indications for spirometry testing.

4. Explain the meaning and importance the following abbreviations during spirometry testing: FVC, FEV_1, FEV_1/FVC ratio.

5. What is the FEV_1/FVC ratio in healthy lungs? What are the ratio ranges used to categorize the extent of COPD?

Exercise 2

 CD-ROM Activity—Preparing the Patient and Performing Spirometry Testing

 30 minutes

- Sign in to Mountain View Clinic.
- From the patient list, select **John R. Simmons**.

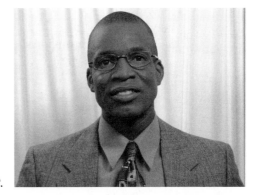

Select John R. Simmons as the patient.

- Highlight and click on **Exam Room** to enter the examination area.

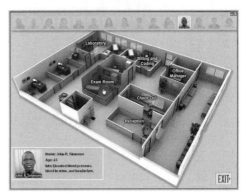

Click on Exam Room.

- Under the Watch heading, click on **Respiratory Testing** to view the video.

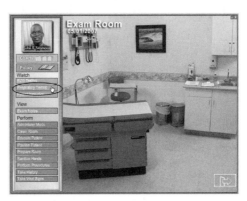

Watch the Respiratory Testing video.

1. What preparation of the patient was provided during the video?

2. During the video, Dr. Simmons asks the medical assistant what the "contraption" is. What would be the proper answer to his question?

3. What other preparation should be given to patients who are coming to the medical office for spirometry testing?

4. What is the proper position for spirometry testing, and why is this important?

5. How many attempts should the patient be given to obtain quality testing?

6. During the testing, what should the medical assistant do to encourage an acceptable test?

➤ • Click **Close** at the end of the video to return to the Exam Room.
 • Click on **Exam Notes** to view the documentation of Dr. Simmons' current visit.

Click on Exam Notes.

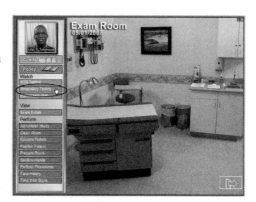

7. Based on your review of the Exam Notes, which of the following patient factors must be taken into account when evaluating spirometry testing? Select all that apply.

_____ Gender

_____ Age

_____ Weight

_____ Body temperature

_____ Blood pressure

_____ Respiratory rate

_____ Height

_____ Heart rate

_____ Time of day

8. True or False:

a. _____ During the video, the medical assistant provided the needed information for Dr. Simmons to obtain an acceptable test.

b. _____ The patient's lips may be loosely pursed around the mouthpiece without affecting the results of the test.

c. _____ The medical assistant should obtain the patient's height and weight before performing the test for computerized spirometers to make the correct calculations.

d. _____ When the test is completed, the mouthpiece may be reused.

e. _____ The medical assistant should provide coaching only while the patient is exhaling air into the mouthpiece.

9. On the blank Progress Notes below, document Dr. Simmons' spirometry testing, including his results of 85%, 90%, and 78% on the peak flow testing.

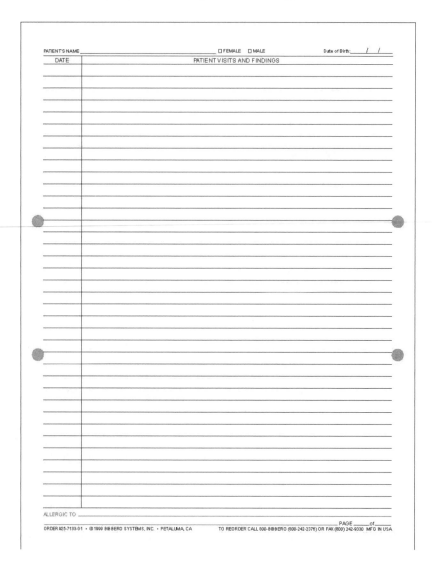

10. Continue reviewing the written documentation of Dr. Simmons' testing in the Exam Notes. Which documentation would be more helpful to the physician?

- Click **Finish** to return to the Exam Room.
- Click the exit arrow to go to the Summary Menu.
- Click **Return to Map** and continue to Exercise 3.

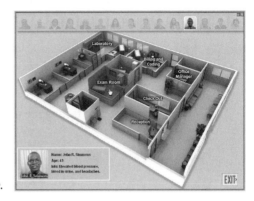

Click Return to Map.

Exercise 3

 CD-ROM Activity—Collecting Sputum Specimens

 15 minutes

- Select **Hu Huang** from the patient list. (*Note:* If you have exited the program, sign in again to Mountain View Clinic and select Hu Huang from the patient list.)

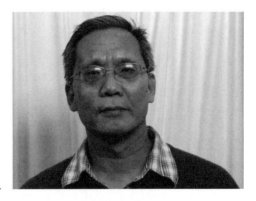

Select Hu Huang.

- On the office map, highlight and click on **Exam Room** to enter the examination area.
- Under Watch, click on **Sputum Collection** to view the video.

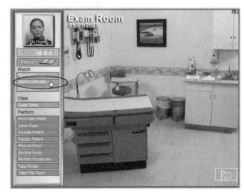

Click on Sputum Collection.

1. What directions should be provided to the patient before obtaining a sputum specimen?

2. Why are sputum specimens usually collected?

3. What types of testing are usually performed on sputum tests?

4. Which of the following PPEs and other supplies are essential for preventing cross contamination when obtaining a sputum specimen? Select all that apply.

_____ Sterile gloves

_____ Gloves

_____ Gown

_____ Goggles/face shield

_____ Shoe covers

_____ Mask

_____ Table covering

_____ Puncture-proof biohazard container

_____ Biohazard waste bag

5. On the blank form below, document the collection of Hu Huang's sputum specimen using today's date, time, and your name.

PATIENT'S NAME	☐ FEMALE ☐ MALE	Date of Birth: / /
DATE	PATIENT VISITS AND FINDINGS	

ALLERGIC TO _____

PAGE ____ of ____

ORDER #25-7133-01 · © 1999 BIBBERO SYSTEMS, INC. · PETALUMA, CA   TO REORDER CALL 800-BIBBERO (800-242-2376) OR FAX (800) 242-9330 MFD IN USA

Specialty Examination and Procedures: Fecal Occult Blood Testing

Reading Assignment: Chapter 28—Specialty Examinations and Procedures

Patient: John R. Simmons

Objectives:

- Discuss the reasons for collecting fecal specimens.
- Describe the patient preparation necessary before collecting specimens for occult blood.
- Discuss the instructions that should be provided to the patient when obtaining a specimen for occult blood.
- Describe the development of the fecal occult test after the specimen has been obtained.
- Identify the possible indications of a positive fecal occult test.
- Describe the need for quality control when obtaining and testing a fecal specimen.

Exercise 1

 CD-ROM Activity—Patient Instruction for Collecting Fecal Specimens

 40 minutes

- Sign in to Mountain View Clinic.
- Select **John R. Simmons** from the patient list.

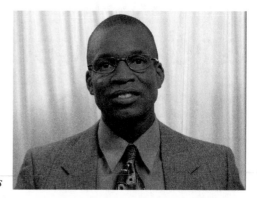

John R. Simmons

- On the office map, highlight and click on **Exam Room** to enter the examination area.

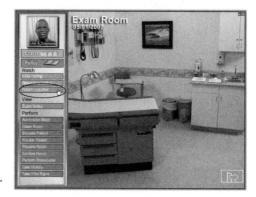

Click on Exam Room.

- Under the Watch heading, select **Patient Instruction** to observe the video.

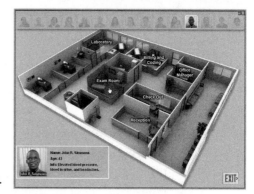

Click on Patient Instruction.

1. Dr. Simmons seems embarrassed by the need to collect stool specimens. How did the medical assistant attempt to put him at ease?

2. Which of the following supplies do patients need in order to obtain fecal specimens at home? Select all that apply.

_____ Gloves

_____ Wooden applicator sticks

_____ Test kits (the number is based on physician's policy)

_____ Plastic wrap

_____ Written instructions

_____ Addressed envelope

3. Which of the following should the medical assistant tell the patient when providing instructions for preparing to obtain a fecal specimen? Select all that apply.

_____ Avoid all vegetables for 3 days.

_____ Eat a high-fiber diet for 2 days.

_____ Eat a meat-free diet for 2 days.

_____ Take all medications ordered by the physician.

_____ Avoid taking aspirin, corticosteroids, and NSAIDs for a week before collecting the specimen.

_____ Do not collect stool specimens during menstrual period or for 3 days afterward.

_____ Eat foods that will cause softening of stools to make the specimen easier to obtain.

_____ Do not eat melons, but eat small amounts of apples, bananas, peaches, and/or pears.

_____ Do not eat turnips, cauliflower, broccoli, or radishes.

_____ Eat vegetables in moderation.

_____ Drink at least three glasses of milk per day.

_____ Do not take iron or vitamin C for 2 days.

_____ Eat moderate amounts of bran cereal, popcorn, and other roughage.

4. When test kits are taken home, how should the patient store the kits until the specimens are collected?

5. What directions should be given to the patient about the timing of specimens?

6. Which of the following are correct instructions to give to the patient about obtaining the stool specimen? Select all that apply.

_____ Using the wooden applicator stick, collect a sample of stool either from a container or from toilet paper.

_____ If the stool falls in the commode, collect the sample as you would from the container or the toilet paper.

_____ Open the flap of the first kit on the left (be sure there are two square boxes inside, labeled A and B); then smear a small amount of stool on the filter paper labeled A, making sure to spread it until thin.

_____ Using the same wooden stick, collect a second sample of stool from another area of the stool.

_____ Place this sample on top of the sample already collected.

_____ Place the second sample in the filter paper box labeled B.

_____ Close the front flap.

_____ Tear this test kit from the other two and place in the envelope provided.

_____ Add the date and time of collection on the flap.

_____ Repeat the same procedure with the next two stools (if three test kits were provided).

_____ Allow the specimens to air-dry before mailing to the office.

_____ Place the specimens in a standard letter-sized envelope and mail.

_____ Place the specimens in an aluminum-lined envelope designed for sending to the medical office.

7. Why is it important that the smear on the test kit be thin?

8. Why is it important that the smears be taken from two different areas of the stool?

9. Why is it important that the patient add roughage to the diet?

10. What is a guaiac test? How is this test related to fecal specimens?

11. On the form below, document the procedure for instructing the patient in collection of a fecal specimen.

PATIENT'S NAME _____ ☐ FEMALE ☐ MALE Date of Birth: __ / __ / __

DATE	PATIENT VISITS AND FINDINGS

ALLERGIC TO _____

ORDER #25-7133-01 • © 1999 BIBBERO SYSTEMS, INC. • PETALUMA, CA   TO REORDER CALL 800-BIBBERO (800-242-2376) OR FAX (800) 242-9330 MFG IN USA   PAGE ____ of ____

Exercise 2

Writing Activity—Developing a Hemoccult Slide Test

20 minutes

A week after his visit, Dr. John R. Simmons has returned the Hemoccult slides to the medical office for development. In this exercise, you will describe the steps necessary to develop the test and provide documentation to the physician.

1. Which of the following are the proper supplies needed for developing the Hemoccult test? Select all that apply.

    _____   Sterile gloves

    _____   Gloves

    _____   Gown and goggles

    _____   Developer solution

    _____   Wooden sticks

    _____   Watch

    _____   Reference card

    _____   Biohazard waste container

    _____   Waste container

2. Now that you have chosen the proper supplies for developing the Hemoccult, match the following columns to show the correct order of steps.

Order	Action
_____ Step 1	a. Ensure quality control by checking the expiration date on slides and developer.
_____ Step 2	b. Don the correct personal protective equipment.
_____ Step 3	c. Dispose of the used Hemoccult slides in proper waste container.
_____ Step 4	
_____ Step 5	d. Read the results in 60 seconds.
_____ Step 6	e. Open the back flap of slides.
_____ Step 7	f. Document the results in the medical record.
_____ Step 8	g. Sanitize hands following procedure.
_____ Step 9	h. Sanitize hands before procedure.
_____ Step 10	i. Compare the results with the reference card.
	j. Apply two drops of developing solution to the guaiac test paper and the quality control area.

3. Why is it important to read the Hemoccult slide results at the end of 60 seconds?

4. What is the volume of fecal blood loss that will result in a positive reading on the Hemoccult test?

5. The result of the first specimen obtained by Dr. Simmons was negative, but slides 2 and 3 were positive. Document these results on the Progress Notes below.

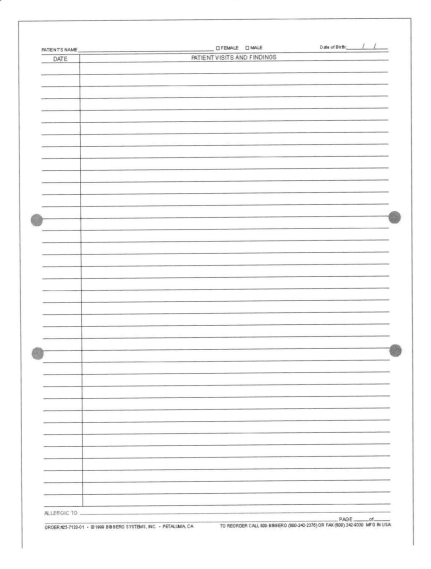

6. What does a positive Hemoccult test indicate?

7. What are the indications if the positive quality control area does not change to a blue color?

8. What are two possible causes of invalid tests?

Urinalysis

👓 **Reading Assignment:** Chapter 30—Urinalysis
- Composition of Urine
- Collection of Urine
- Analysis of Urine

Patient: Janet Jones

Objectives:

- Discuss the reasons for performing urinalysis.
- Explain the different means of collecting urine specimens.
- Describe the differences in testing results that can be expected with random and clean-catch midstream specimens.
- Describe the procedure for performing a dipstick urine specimen.
- Discuss the composition of urine.
- Prepare a laboratory requisition for a dipstick urinalysis.
- Discuss the determinants in the physical examination of urine.
- Explain the differences between qualitative and quantitative testing of urine.
- Describe the steps in quality control with urine testing.

Exercise 1

Writing Activity—Urine Components and Collection

 25 minutes

   1. On the diagram below, label the organs of the urinary tract.

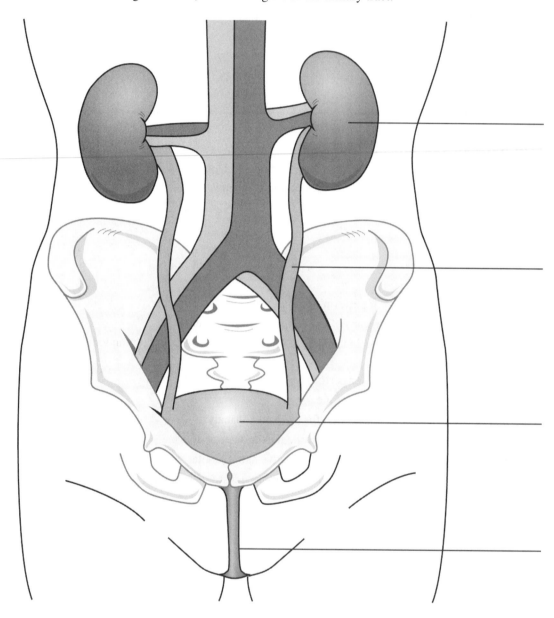

   2. Which of the following are valid reasons for performing urinalyses?
     a. For assessment of pathologic conditions in body systems
     b. As a screening measure for the possibility of pathologic conditions
     c. To assist in evaluation of the effectiveness of medical treatment
     d. For detection of abused substances
     e. All of the above

3. Which of the following are urine collection methods used routinely in the medical office? Select all that apply.

_____ Random samples

_____ Last-voided specimen of the day

_____ 24-hour urine specimens

_____ Clean-catch midstream specimen

_____ Catheterized specimens

_____ Early-morning voided specimens

_____ First-voided morning specimens

_____ Sterile specimens

4. Which of the following are important guidelines in collecting a urine specimen? Select all that apply.

_____ Obtain a full cup of urine.

_____ Obtain 30-50 mL of urine.

_____ Label the specimen with the patient's name only.

_____ Label the specimen with the patient's name and the date and time of collection.

_____ Label the specimen with the patient's name, the date and time of collection, and the type of specimen.

_____ Label the specimen with the patient's name, the date and time of collection, and the initials of the person handling the specimen.

_____ Medications should be recorded on the lab requisition.

_____ Collection of urine should be avoided during menstruation.

_____ The medical assistant should allow time for the patient to void and supply water for the patient to drink if necessary.

_____ The medical assistant should not allow the patient to leave the office until the specimen has been collected.

5. What instructions should be given to the patient for a 24-hour urine specimen?

Exercise 2

  CD-ROM Activity—Performing a Urinalysis

 25 minutes

1. What differences in test results could be expected with random catch and clean-catch mid-stream urine specimens?

> • Sign in to Mountain View Clinic.
> • From the patient list, select **Janet Jones**.

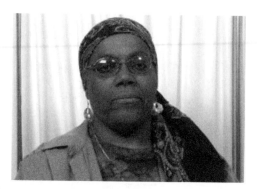

Select Janet Jones.

• On the office map, highlight and click on **Exam Room**.

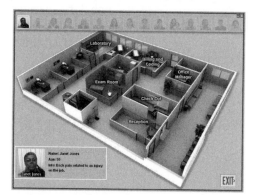

Click on Exam Room.

• Under the Watch heading, select **Specimen Collection** to view the video.

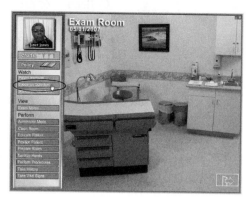

Click on Specimen Collection.

- At the end of the video, click **Close**. Then click on the exit arrow to go to the Summary Menu.
- Click on **Return to Map**.

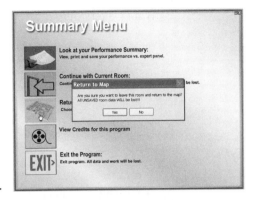

Click on Return to Map.

- From the office map, highlight and click on **Billing and Coding**.

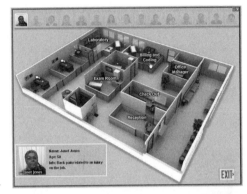

Click on Billing and Coding.

- Click on **Charts** to open Ms. Jones' medical record.

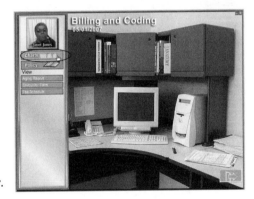

Click on Charts.

- When the chart opens, click on the **Workers' Comp** tab. Then select **2-Progress Notes** from the drop-down menu.
- Review Ms. Jones' Progress Notes, specifically watching for data regarding her previous medical history.

2. Why would it be important for Ms. Jones to provide a urine specimen, based on her medical history?

3. What is ureterolithiasis?

4. The three components of a urinalysis are _____,

   _____, and _____ analysis of the urine.

5. In a urinalysis, what four physical properties should be determined?

6. Which of the following are valid terms for describing the appearance of urine? Select all that apply.

   _____ Clear

   _____ Smokey

   _____ Bright

   _____ Cloudy

   _____ Heavily cloudy

   _____ Slightly cloudy

   _____ Very cloudy

   _____ OK

7. Which of the following are *incorrect* terms for describing the color of urine? Select all that apply.

   _____ Straw

   _____ Orange

   _____ Yellow

   _____ Light and dark straw

   _____ Brownish red

   _____ Amber

   _____ Dark yellow

8. What are some of the causes of odoriferous urine?

9. Urine should have a slightly _____ odor.

10. True or False:

   a. _____ Cloudiness of urine is always a sign that the urine contains bacteria.

   b. _____ Urine should be tested as soon as possible after collection.

   c. _____ The smell of ammonia may be an indication of a UTI.

   d. _____ The color of urine is caused by urochrome from the breakdown of hemoglobin.

   e. _____ The color of urine may vary from dark yellow to almost colorless.

   f. _____ A milky appearance of urine may be caused by fat droplets or pus.

   g. _____ Blood is always apparent in urine when present.

   h. _____ Drugs do not have any effect on the color of urine.

   i. _____ A musty smell to urine may come from foods eaten.

   j. _____ A fruity odor to urine may be a sign of diabetes.

   k. _____ The longer urine stands after collection, the more likely bacteria are to grow.

   l. _____ The specific gravity of urine measures the weight of urine compared with water.

11. Do you think that the medical assistant in the video was professional in providing information to Ms. Jones? Support your answer.

12. Other than the patient's past history, what medical reason would Dr. Meyer have for obtaining a urine specimen from Ms. Jones?

13. When the chemical examination of urine is measured in amounts such as 1+, 2+, etc., this is

    considered a _____ (**qualitative** or **quantitative**) testing of urine.

14. When chemical examination of urine is reported in measurable units such as mg/dL, the test

    is reported as a _____ (**qualitative** or **quantitative**) test.

15. Which of the following can be found on a dipstick urine test? Select all that apply.

    _____ Protein

    _____ Alcohol

    _____ Blood

    _____ White blood cells

    _____ Glucose/ketones

    _____ Urobilinogen

    _____ Bile

    _____ Bilirubin

    _____ Nitrite

    _____ pH

    _____ Acidity/alkalinity

    _____ Specific gravity

    _____ Color

16. Which of the following are proper guidelines for using reagent strips for urine testing?
    Select all that apply.

    _____ The specimen should be freshly voided.

    _____ Reagent strips may be used only with a clean-catch midstream specimen.

    _____ The specimen container should be clean and dry.

    _____ The container should be free of detergent.

    _____ The container must be sterile.

    _____ First-voided morning specimens provide the best results for all tests.

    _____ Specimens should be read against the color card for the test.

    _____ The amount of lighting available when reading the test is not important.

    _____ Reagent strips may be stored under any conditions.

_____ The desiccant in the specimen bottle should remain in place until all strips have been used.

_____ Reagent strips are best when stored in the refrigerator.

_____ Discoloration of the strips has no effect on testing.

_____ Quality control on the strips should be performed each day.

_____ Quality control ensures reliability of the test results.

17. True or False:

a. _____ Microscopic examination of urine specimens is a CLIA-waived test.

b. _____ Red blood cells in urine are easily seen under a microscope.

c. _____ White blood cells are larger than red blood cells and are more easily seen.

d. _____ Epithelial cells in urine are the result of sloughing of the outer layer of skin.

e. _____ Squamous epithelial cells are not uncommon in urine specimens of females.

f. _____ Renal epithelial cells are considered normal in a urine specimen.

g. _____ Various crystals and casts may be found in urine.

h. _____ Drugs may produce crystals in urine.

18. On the blank Progress Notes below, document the following urine specimen testing results for Janet Jones (using today's date and time):
   - The dipstick urine is albumin 1+, glucose 3+, leukocytes moderate, and 5-7/hpf.
   - The color is amber, and the physical appearance is cloudy.
   - Some fat droplets and powder crystals are seen.
   - All other results are negative.

PATIENT'S NAME	☐ FEMALE ☐ MALE	Date of Birth: __/__/__
DATE	PATIENT VISITS AND FINDINGS	

ALLERGIC TO _____

ORDER #25-7133-01 • © 1999 BIBBERO SYSTEMS, INC. • PETALUMA, CA   TO REORDER CALL 800-BIBBERO (800-242-2376) OR FAX (800) 242-9330 MFG IN USA   PAGE ____ of ____

19. If Dr. Meyer believed it was necessary, she could have ordered a random urine specimen for Ms. Jones to be sent to the lab for routine urinalysis with a microscopic and quantitative analysis. Prepare the lab requisition form below to order this test for the patient (using today's date and the time of her appointment).

Lab Services

IMPORTANT
Patient instructions
and map on back

PHYSICIAN ORDERS

M ☐ Patient
F ☐ SS# _____ – ____ – ____

Patient _____ _____ D.O.B. _____
        Last Name   First   M.I.

Address _____ City _____ Zip _____ Phone # _____

Physician _____
ATTACH COPY OF INSURANCE CARD

Date & Time of Collection:
_____ _____

Drawing Facility: _____

Diagnosis/ICD-9 Code _____
(Additional codes on reverse)

☐ 789.00 Abdominal Pain
☐ 285.9 Anemia (NOS)
☐ 414.9 Coronary Artery Disease (CAD)
☐ 250.0 DM (diabetes mellitus)
☐ 780.7 Fatigue/Malaise
☐ 272.0 Hypercholesterolemia
☐ 244.9 Hypothyroidism
☐ 272.4 Hyperlipidemia
☐ 401.9 Hypertension
☐ 485.9 URI (upper respiratory infection)

☐ ROUTINE
☐ ASAP
☐ STAT

☐ PHONE RESULTS TO: # _____
☐ FAX RESULTS TO: # _____
☐ COPY TO: _____

HEMATOLOGY

☐ 1021 CBC, Automated Diff (incl. Platelet Ct.)
☐ 1023 Hemoglobin/Hematocrit
☐ 1020 Hemogram
☐ 1025 Platelet Count
☐ 1150 Pro Time Diagnostic
☐ 1151 Pro Time, Therapeutic
☐ 1155 PTT
☐ 1315 Reticulocyte Count
☐ 1310 Sed Rate/Westergren

URINE

☐ 1059 Urinalysis
☐ 1082 Urinalysis w/Culture if indicated
    Urine-24 Hr _____ Spot _____
    Ht. _____ Wt. _____
☐ 3033 Creatinine
☐ 3036 Creatinine Clearance (also requires blood)
☐ 3398 Protein
☐ 3096 Sodium/Potassium
☐ Microalbumin 24 Hr _____ Spot _____

SEROLOGY

☐ 8020 ANA (Antinuclear Antibody)
☐ 8040 Mono Spot
☐ 3494 Rheumatoid Factor
☐ 8010 RPR
☐ 5365 Rubella

CHEMISTRY

☐ 5550 Alpha Fetoprotein, Prenatal
☐ 3000 Amylase
☐ 3153 B12/Folate
☐ 3156 Beta HCG, Quantitative
☐ 3321 Bilirubin, Total
☐ 3324 Bilirubin, Total/Direct
☐ 3009 BUN
☐ 3159 CEA
☐ 3348 Cholesterol
☐ 3030 Creatinine, Serum
☐ 3509 Digoxin (recommend 12 hrs., after dose)
☐ 3515 Dilantin
☐ 3168 Ferritin
☐ 3193 FSH
☐ 3066 ▼ Glucose, Fasting
☐ 3061 ▼ Glucose, 1° Post 50 g Glucola
☐ 3075 ▼ Glucose, 2° Post Glucola
☐ 3060 Glucose, 2° Post Prandial (meal)
☐ 3049 ▼ Glucose Tolerance Oral GTT
☐ 3047 ▼ Glucose Tolerance Gestational GTT
☐ 3650 Hemoglobin, A1C

CHEMISTRY

☐ 5232 HBsAg
☐ 3175 HIV (Consent required)
☐ 3581 Iron & Iron Binding Capacity
☐ 3195 LH
☐ 3590 Magnesium
☐ 3527 Phenobarbital
☐ 3095 Potassium
☐ 3689 Pregnancy Test, Serum (HCG, qual)
☐ 3653 Pregnancy Test, Urine
☐ 3197 Prolactin
☐ 3199 PSA
☐ 3339 SGOT/AST
☐ 3342 SGPT/ALT
☐ 3093 Sodium/Potassium, Serum
☐ 3510 Tegretol
☐ 3551 Theophylline
☐ 3333 Uric Acid

MICROBIOLOGY

Source _____
☐ 7240 Culture, AFB
☐ 7200 Culture, Blood x _____
☐ Draw Interval _____
☐ 7280 Culture, Fungus
☐ Culture, Routine
☐ 7005 Culture, Stool
☐ 7010 Culture, Throat
☐ 7000 Culture, Urine
☐ 7300 Gram Stain
☐ 7355 Occult Blood x _____
☐ 7365 Ova & Parasites x _____
☐ 7400 Smear & Suspension
    (includes Gram Stain/Wet Mount)
☐ 7060 Rapid Strep A Screen (Negs confir by cult)
☐ 7065 Rapid Strep A Screen only
☐ 7030 Beta Strep Culture
☐ 5207 GC by DNA Probe
☐ 5130 Chlamydia by DNA Probe
☐ 5555 Chlamydia/GC by DNA Probe
☐ 7375 Wright Stain, Stool

Additional Tests _____

PANELS & PROFILES

☐ X **3309 CHEM 12**
Albumin, Alkaline Phosphatase, BUN, Calcium, Cholesterol, Glucose, LDH, Phosphorus, AST, Total Bilirubin, Total Protein, Uric Acid

☐ ▼ **3315 CHEM 20**
Chem 12, Electrolyte Panel, Creatinine, Iron, Gamma GT, ALT, Triglycerides

☐ ▼ **3357 CARDIAC RISK PANEL**
Cholesterol, HDL, LDL, Risk Factors, VLDL, Triglycerides

☐ X **3042 CRITICAL CARE PANEL**
BUN, Chloride, CO2, Glucose, Potassium, Sodium

☐ **3046 ELECTROLYTE PANEL**
Chloride, CO2, Potassium, Sodium

☐ ▼ **3399 EXECUTIVE PANEL**
Chem 20, Iron, Cardiac Risk Panel, CBC, RPR, Thyroid Cascade

☐ **5242 HEPATITIS PANEL, ACUTE**
HAVIgMAb, HBsAg, HBsAb, HBcAb, HCVAb

☐ ▼ **3355 LIPID MONITORING PANEL**
Cholesterol, Triglycerides, HDL, LDL, VLDL, ALT, AST

☐ **3312 LIVER PANEL**
Alkaline Phosphatase, AST, Total Bilirubin, Gamma GT, Total Protein, Albumin, ALT

☐ X **3083 METABOLIC STATUS PANEL**
BUN, Osmolality (calculated), Chloride, CO2, Creatinine, Glucose, Potassium, Sodium, BUN/Creatinine, Ratio, Anion Gap

☐ X **3376 PANEL B**
Chem 12, CBC, Electrolyte Panel

☐ ▼ **3382 PANEL D**
Chem 20, CBC, Thyroid Cascade

☐ X **3388 PANEL F**
Chem 12, CBC, Electrolyte Panel, Thyroid Cascade

☐ ▼ **3391 PANEL G**
Chem 20, Cardiac Risk Panel, CBC, Thyroid Cascade

☐ ▼ **3393 PANEL H**
Chem 20, CBC, Cardiac Risk Panel Rheumatoid Factor, Thyroid Cascade

☐ ▼ **3397 PANEL J**
Chem 20, Cardiac Risk Panel

☐ **5351 PRENATAL PANEL**
Antibody Screen ABO/Rh, CBC, Rubella, HBsAg, RPR
☐ 1059 with Urinalysis, Routine
☐ 1082 with Urinalysis w/Culture if indicated

☐ X **3102 RENAL PANEL**
Metabolic Status Panel, Calcium, Phosphorus

☐ **3188 THYROID CASCADE**
TSH, Reflex Testing

▼ - patient **required** to fast for 12-14 hours

X - patient **recommended** to fast 12-14 hours

LAB USE ONLY   INIT _____
☐ SST   ☐ PLASMA
☐ PURPLE   ☐ SERUM
☐ YELLOW   ☐ SWAB
☐ BLUE   ☐ SLIDES
☐ GREEN   ☐ DNA PROBE
☐ GREY   ☐ B. CULT BTLS
☐ URINE
☐ BLACK
☐ OTHER: _____
REC'V. SPECIMEN: ☐ FROZEN
☐ AMBIENT   ☐ ON ICE

Special Instructions/Pertinent Clinical Information _____

Physician's Signature _____   Date _____

These orders may be FAXed to: 449-5288

7060-500 (7/96)

LAB

Clean-Catch Urine

👓 **Reading Assignment:** Chapter 30—Urinalysis
- Urine Pregnancy Testing

Patient: Louise Parlet

Objectives:

- Discuss the reason for obtaining clean-catch midstream urine specimens.
- Describe the instructions needed to prepare a patient, either male or female, for obtaining a clean-catch midstream urine specimen.
- Discuss how breaks in proper technique can lead to possible errors in diagnoses.

Exercise 1

CD-ROM Activity—Patient Education for
Clean-Catch Midstream Urine Collection

 30 minutes

1. Why is it so important to provide proper patient education about the correct collection method for obtaining a clean-catch midstream urine specimen?

2. True or False:

   a. _____ All urine specimens collected in the medical office must be clean-catch midstream samples.

   b. _____ The container used to obtain a clean-catch midstream urine sample must be aseptically clean.

   c. _____ The clean-catch midstream procedure requires the patient to follow specific instructions when obtaining the specimen.

   d. _____ A clean-catch midstream urine sample is used to check for urinary tract infections.

   e. _____ The patient has responsibility in the proper collection of the specimen.

   f. _____ Before collecting the specimen, a female patient should cleanse the perineum from back to front.

   g. _____ Before collecting the specimen, a male patient should cleanse the head of the penis in a circular motion from the urethral opening outward.

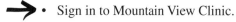 • Sign in to Mountain View Clinic.
 • Select **Louise Parlet** from the patient list.

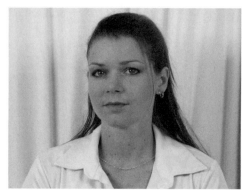

Louise Parlet

➤ • On the office map, click on **Exam Room**.

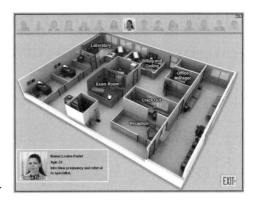

Go to the Exam Room.

• Under the Watch heading, select **Urine Specimen Collection** to view the video.

3. In the video, the medical assistant provided information that is not correct. What incorrect information was given to the patient? What is the correct instruction?

➤ • Next, under the Perform heading, click on **Prepare Room**.

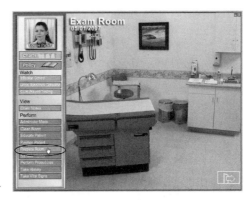

Click on Prepare Room.

• Begin choosing the supplies needed for Louise Parlet's visit. (*Note:* You can reopen the Exam Notes for reference as you make your selections.)

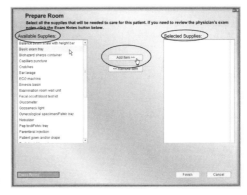

Select the supplies needed for this visit.

- Repeat this step until you are satisfied you have everything you need from the list.
- After completing your selections, click **Finish** to return to the Exam Room.

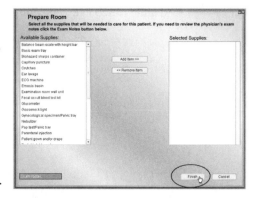

Click Finish to return to the Exam Room.

- Click the exit arrow to go to the Summary Menu.
- Click on **Look at Your Performance Summary**. Scroll down to the Prepare Room section to compare your answers with those of the experts. This summary can also be printed or saved for your instructor.

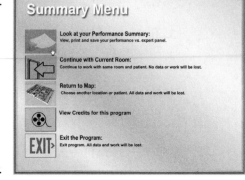

Click on Look at Your Performance Summary.

- Click on **Close** to return to the Summary Menu.
- Click on **Return to Map**.

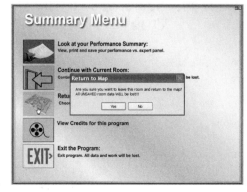

Click on Return to Map.

4. Match the following columns to show the correct order of steps in the collection of a clean-catch midstream urine specimen.

Order	Action
_____ Step 1	a. Clean the sides of the perineum or the head of the penis.
_____ Step 2	b. Wash hands.
_____ Step 3	c. Cleanse the middle of the perineum or the head of the penis.
_____ Step 4	d. Complete voiding (not into the container).
_____ Step 5	e. Void a small amount of urine, not catching the urine in the container.
_____ Step 6	
	f. Void into the container.
_____ Step 7	
	g. Hold the container without touching the rim.
_____ Step 8	
	h. Hold open the labia of the female with one hand or retract the foreskin on the male if necessary.
_____ Step 9	
_____ Step 10	i. Open collection container without touching the rim or inside.
	j. Close container, taking care to not touch rim or inside.

5. Why is it important that the patient be reminded to wash his or her hands before obtaining the specimen?

6. What are some of the possible problems that may be encountered if the patient is not properly prepared for obtaining the urine specimen?

7. After the specimen has been collected, how long should it be allowed to stand prior to testing?

8. Which of the following should be included in charting the collection a clean-catch midstream urine specimen? Select all that apply.

_____ Date of collection

_____ Time of collection

_____ Time that the specimen was provided to the lab

_____ Type of specimen collected

_____ Instructions provided to the patient

_____ Type of test ordered

_____ Signature of person doing the charting

→ • On the office map, highlight and click on **Laboratory**.

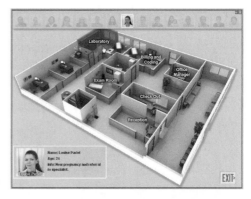

Click on Laboratory.

• Under the Perform heading, click on **Collect Specimens**.

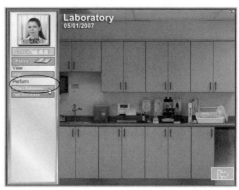

Click on Collect Specimens.

→ • Next, select all the tests ordered for Louise Parlet that require urine collection. (*Note:* If you wish to review the notes for this visit, click on **Charts** and select **3-Progress Notes** from the menu under the **Patient Medical Information** tab.)

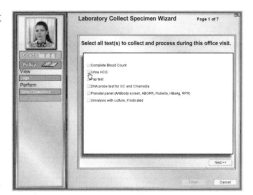

Select the tests requiring urine collection.

• A series of questions will be asked for each test you selected. Answer all the questions related to each test; then click **Finish** to return to the Laboratory. (*Remember:* The Policy Manual can be opened at any time for reference as you answer the questions.)

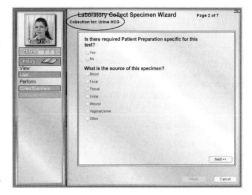

Answer the questions for each selected test.

• Click on **Charts** and then on the **Patient Medical Information** tab. Select **3-Progress Notes** from the drop-down menu. Review as needed to complete the form in question 9.

9. Below, complete the lab requisition form as ordered in the Progress Notes by Dr. Hayler.

Lab Services

IMPORTANT
Patient instructions
and map on back

PHYSICIAN ORDERS

M ☐ Patient
F ☐ SS# ___ – ___ – ___

Patient _____ _____ ___ D.O.B. _____
Last Name   First   M.I.

Address _____ City _____ Zip _____ Phone # _____

Physician _____
ATTACH COPY OF INSURANCE CARD

Date & Time of Collection:
_____ _____

Drawing
Facility: _____

Diagnosis/ICD-9 Code _____
(Additional codes on reverse)

☐ ROUTINE ☐ PHONE RESULTS TO: # _____
☐ ASAP   ☐ FAX RESULTS TO: # _____
☐ STAT   ☐ COPY TO: _____

☐ 789.00 Abdominal Pain
☐ 285.9 Anemia (NOS)
☐ 414.9 Coronary Artery Disease (CAD)
☐ 250.0 DM (diabetes mellitus)
☐ 780.7 Fatigue/Malaise
☐ 272.0 Hypercholesterolemia
☐ 244.9 Hypothyroidism
☐ 272.4 Hyperlipidemia
☐ 401.9 Hypertension
☐ 485.9 URI (upper respiratory infection)

HEMATOLOGY	CHEMISTRY	CHEMISTRY	MICROBIOLOGY
☐ 1021 CBC, Automated Diff (incl. Platelet Ct.)	☐ 5550 Alpha Fetoprotein, Prenatal	☐ 5232 HBsAg	
☐ 1023 Hemoglobin/Hematocrit	☐ 3000 Amylase	☐ 3175 HIV (Consent required)	Source _____
☐ 1020 Hemogram	☐ 3153 B12/Folate	☐ 3581 Iron & Iron Binding Capacity	☐ 7240 Culture, AFB
☐ 1025 Platelet Count	☐ 3156 Beta HCG, Quantitative	☐ 3195 LH	☐ 7200 Culture, Blood x _____
☐ 1150 Pro Time Diagnostic	☐ 3321 Bilirubin, Total	☐ 3590 Magnesium	☐ Draw Interval _____
☐ 1151 Pro Time, Therapeutic	☐ 3324 Bilirubin, Total/Direct	☐ 3527 Phenobarbital	☐ 7280 Culture, Fungus
☐ 1155 PTT	☐ 3009 BUN	☐ 3095 Potassium	☐ Culture, Routine
☐ 1315 Reticulocyte Count	☐ 3159 CEA	☐ 3689 Pregnancy Test, Serum (HCG, qual)	☐ 7005 Culture, Stool
☐ 1310 Sed Rate/Westergren	☐ 3348 Cholesterol	☐ 3653 Pregnancy Test, Urine	☐ 7010 Culture, Throat
	☐ 3030 Creatinine, Serum	☐ 3197 Prolactin	☐ 7000 Culture, Urine
URINE	☐ 3509 Digoxin (recommend 12 hrs., after dose)	☐ 3199 PSA	☐ 7300 Gram Stain
☐ 1059 Urinalysis	☐ 3515 Dilantin	☐ 3339 SGOT/AST	☐ 7355 Occult Blood x _____
☐ 1082 Urinalysis w/Culture if indicated	☐ 3168 Ferritin	☐ 3342 SGPT/ALT	☐ 7365 Ova & Parasites x _____
Urine-24 Hr _____ Spot _____	☐ 3193 FSH	☐ 3093 Sodium/Potassium, Serum	☐ 7400 Smear & Suspension
Ht. _____ Wt. _____	☐ 3066 ▼ Glucose, Fasting	☐ 3510 Tegretol	(includes Gram Stain/Wet Mount)
☐ 3033 Creatinine	☐ 3061 Glucose, 1° Post 50 g Glucola	☐ 3551 Theophylline	☐ 7060 Rapid Strep A Screen (Negs confir by cult)
☐ 3036 Creatinine Clearance (also requires blood)	☐ 3075 ▼ Glucose, 2° Post Glucola	☐ 3333 Uric Acid	☐ 7065 Rapid Strep A Screen only
☐ 3398 Protein	☐ 3060 ▼ Glucose, 2° Post Prandial (meal)		☐ 7030 Beta Strep Culture
☐ 3096 Sodium/Potassium	☐ 3049 ▼ Glucose Tolerance Oral GTT		☐ 5207 GC by DNA Probe
☐ Microalbumin 24 Hr _____ Spot _____	☐ 3047 ▼Glucose Tolerance Gestational GTT		☐ 5130 Chlamydia by DNA Probe
SEROLOGY	☐ 3650 Hemoglobin, A1C		☐ 5555 Chlamydia/GC by DNA Probe
☐ 8020 ANA (Antinuclear Antibody)			☐ 7375 Wright Stain, Stool
☐ 8040 Mono Spot			
☐ 3494 Rheumatoid Factor			
☐ 8010 RPR			
☐ 5365 Rubella	Additional Tests _____		

PANELS & PROFILES

☐ X **3309 CHEM 12**
Albumin, Alkaline Phosphatase, BUN, Calcium, Cholesterol, Glucose, LDH, Phosphorus, AST, Total Bilirubin, Total Protein, Uric Acid

☐ ▼ **3315 CHEM 20**
Chem 12, Electrolyte Panel, Creatinine, Iron, Gamma GT, ALT, Triglycerides

☐ ▼ **3357 CARDIAC RISK PANEL**
Cholesterol, HDL, LDL, Risk Factors, VLDL Triglycerides

☐ X **3042 CRITICAL CARE PANEL**
BUN, Chloride, CO2, Glucose, Potassium, Sodium

☐ **3046 ELECTROLYTE PANEL**
Chloride, CO2, Potassium, Sodium

☐ ▼ **3399 EXECUTIVE PANEL**
Chem 20, Iron, Cardiac Risk Panel, CBC, RPR, Thyroid Cascade

☐ **5242 HEPATITIS PANEL, ACUTE**
HAVIgMAb, HBsAg, HBsAb, HBcAb, HCVAb

☐ ▼ **3355 LIPID MONITORING PANEL**
Cholesterol, Triglycerides, HDL, LDL, VLDL, ALT, AST

☐ **3312 LIVER PANEL**
Alkaline Phospatase, AST, Total Bilirubin, Gamma GT, Total Protein, Albumin, ALT

☐ X **3083 METABOLIC STATUS PANEL**
BUN, Osmolality (calculated), Chloride, CO2 Creatinine, Glucose, Potassium, Sodium, BUN/Creatinine, Ratio, Anion Gap

☐ X **3376 PANEL B**
Chem 12, CBC, Electrolyte Panel

☐ ▼ **3382 PANEL D**
Chem 20, CBC, Thyroid Cascade

☐ X **3386 PANEL F**
Chem 12, CBC, Electrolyte Panel, Thyroid Cascade

☐ ▼ **3391 PANEL G**
Chem 20, Cardiac Risk Panel, CBC, Thyroid Cascade

☐ ▼ **3393 PANEL H**
Chem 20, CBC, Cardiac Risk Panel Rheumatoid Factor, Thyroid Cascade

☐ ▼ **3397 PANEL J**
Chem 20, Cardiac Risk Panel

☐ **5351 PRENATAL PANEL**
Antibody Screen ABO/Rh, CBC Rubella, HBsAg, RPR
☐ 1059 with Urinalysis, Routine
☐ 1082 with Urinalysis w/Culture if indicated

☐ X **3102 RENAL PANEL**
Metabolic Status Panel, Calcium, Phosphorus

☐ **3188 THYROID CASCADE**
TSH, Reflex Testing

▼ - patient **required** to fast for 12-14 hours

X - patient recommended to fast 12-14 hours

LAB USE ONLY	INIT _____
☐ SST	☐ PLASMA
☐ PURPLE	☐ SERUM
☐ YELLOW	☐ SWAB
☐ BLUE	☐ SLIDES
☐ GREEN	☐ DNA PROBE
☐ GREY	☐ B. CULT BTLS
☐ URINE	
☐ BLACK	
☐ OTHER: _____	
REC'V. SPECIMEN:	☐ FROZEN
☐ AMBIENT	☐ ON ICE

Special Instructions/Pertinent Clinical Information _____

Physician's Signature _____   **Date** _____

These orders may be FAXed to: 449-5288

7060-500 (7/96)

LAB

10. Note that a urine culture can be ordered in two different places on the lab requisition. What is the difference between the two?

Phlebotomy

Reading Assignment: Chapter 29—Introduction to the Clinical Laboratory
Chapter 31—Phlebotomy

Patient: Kevin McKinzie

Objectives:

- Identify the most commonly used venipuncture sites.
- Identify the types of specimens that can be obtained by venipuncture.
- Discuss the necessary preparation of the patient for a routine venipuncture.
- Determine what supplies are needed for a venipuncture.
- Review the need for OSHA standards and standard precautions with venipuncture.
- Understand why proper positioning of the patient for venipuncture is necessary.
- Identify the process for safe capillary puncture on infants and older children or adults.
- Describe equipment and supplies needed for capillary puncture.

Exercise 1

 CD-ROM Activity—Identifying the Necessary Supplies for Venipuncture

 20 minutes

- Sign in to Mountain View Clinic.
- Select **Kevin McKinzie** from the patient list.

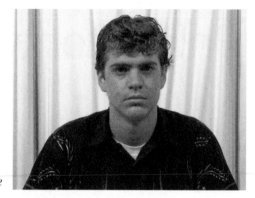

Kevin McKinzie

- On the office map, click on **Exam Room**. Next, select **Exam Notes** to review the notes for the current visit.

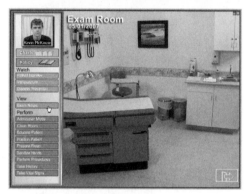

In the Exam Room, click on Exam Notes.

- Read the Exam Notes, making note of the blood tests that will require phlebotomy during this visit.
- Click **Finish** to close the Exam Notes.
- Now select **Prepare Room** (under Perform) to choose the supplies and equipment needed for Kevin McKinzie's visit.

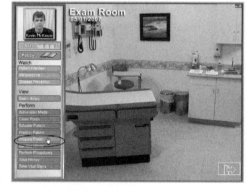

Select Prepare Room.

- From the alphabetical list, select the first item needed for this visit; then click **Add Item** to confirm your choice. The items you select will appear in the Selected Supplies column.
- Repeat this step until you have everything you need from the list. (*Hint:* The Exam Notes are available if you need to refer to them.)

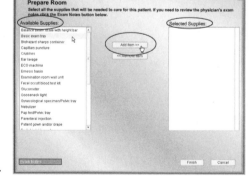

Select the supplies needed for this visit.

- After completing your selections, click **Finish** to return to the Exam Room.

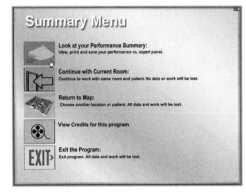

Click Finish to return to the Exam Room.

- Click the exit arrow to go to the Summary Menu.
- Click on **Look at Your Performance Summary**. Scroll down to the Prepare Room section to compare your answers with those of the experts. This summary can be printed or saved for your instructor.

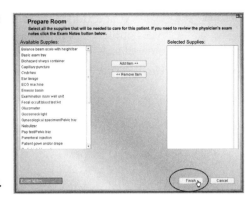

Click on Look at Your Performance Summary.

- Click on **Close** and then on **Return to Map**.

1. Which of the following tests will require blood for completion of the physician's orders for the visit? Select all that apply.

   _____ Urinalysis

   _____ CBC with differential

   _____ Hepatitis panel

   _____ Liver panel

   _____ EBV antibody

   _____ MonoSpot test

2. Which of the tests you selected in question 1 would be sent to an outside lab for testing?

- Using your textbook for reference, decide what types of blood specimens will be needed for the ordered tests.
- On the office map, click to enter the **Laboratory**.

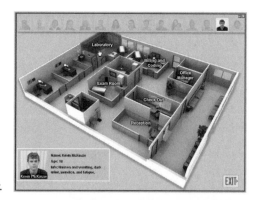

Click on Laboratory.

- Under Perform, select **Collect Specimens**.

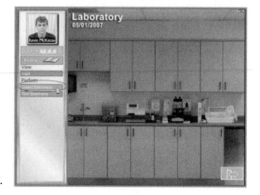

Click on Collect Specimens.

- Next, select all the tests that require blood collection. (*Hint:* To review the notes for the visit, click on **Charts** and select **1-Progress Notes** under the **Patient Medical Information** tab.)

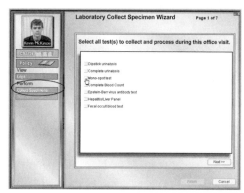

Select all the required blood tests.

- A series of questions will be asked for each test you selected. Answer all the questions related to each test; then click **Finish** to return to the Laboratory. (*Hint:* The Policy Manual can be opened for reference as you answer the questions.)

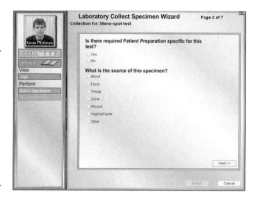

Answer the questions for each selected test.

- Click the exit arrow to return to the Summary Menu.
- Select **Look at Your Performance Summary** to check your answers with the experts.
- Expert responses are given separately for each test. Scroll down to locate the test you want to review. Your summary can be printed or saved for your instructor.

3. True or False:

   a. _____ Serum is obtained from whole blood that is centrifuged immediately after collection.

   b. _____ Plasma is obtained from whole blood that has an anticoagulant added to the test tube to prevent clotting.

   c. _____ Whole blood is needed for a CBC with differential.

   d. _____ Serum is needed for the hepatitis panel and the liver panel.

   e. _____ Serum contains the chemicals found in the blood with the clotting factors removed.

   f. _____ Plasma contains the chemicals found in the blood with the clotting factors removed.

   g. _____ Evacuated tubes are available in only one size.

   h. _____ Evacuated tubes have an expiration date and a label for writing the patient name.

   i. _____ The needle within the Vacutainer should be pierced after the needle has entered the vein.

   j. _____ If the top of the evacuated tube will need to be opened, a Hemoguard tube should be used.

   k. _____ Before using an evacuated tube, you should check it for cracks and other breaches in quality control.

   l. _____ If a Vacutainer tube is dropped, it can still be used unless it is cracked or broken.

   m. _____ The evacuated tube should be filled to the level of blood specified for the test, not to the size of the tube.

   n. _____ Tubes containing additives should be agitated 8 to 10 times to mix the blood with the additive.

4. Serum can be collected in _____ or _____ tubes that contain no additives.

5. List the parts of the Vacutainer system.

6. Match the columns below to indicate the correct order of tubes to be used when drawing blood for testing.

Order	Tube Stopper Color
_____ 1st	a. Lavender top
_____ 2nd	b. Yellow top or sterile tube for blood cultures
_____ 3rd	c. Red top or speckled top for serum
_____ 4th	d. Gray top
_____ 5th	e. Light blue top for coagulation studies
_____ 6th	f. Green top

• Click on **Close** and then on **Return to Map**.
• Click on **Exam Room** and continue to Exercise 2.

Exercise 2

 CD-ROM Activity—Choosing the Correct Position and Site for a Venipuncture

 15 minutes

- In this exercise we will continue with Kevin McKinzie's visit. (*Note:* If you have exited the program, sign in again to Mountain View Clinic, select Kevin McKinzie, and go to the Exam Room.)

    1. As a medical assistant, you will decide on the proper site for venipuncture. On the figures below, label the venipuncture sites that are most appropriate for obtaining blood specimens.

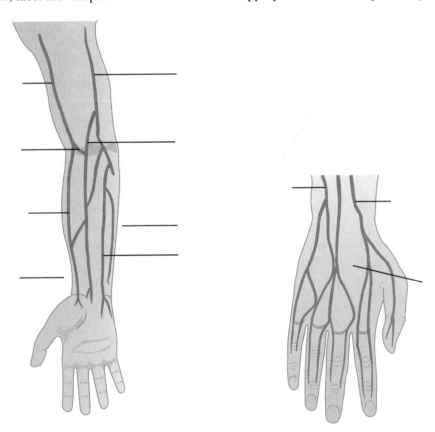

    2. What are the advantages of using the veins found in the antecubital fossa?

    3. If the veins are not easily palpable, what should be the next step in venipuncture?

➡ • On the office map, click on **Exam Room**.

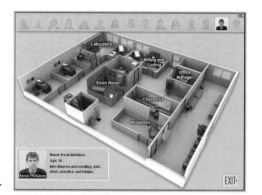

Click on Exam Room.

• From the Exam Room menu, select **Venipuncture** and watch the video.

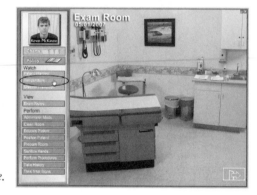

Click on Venipuncture.

• At the end of the video, click **Close** to return to the Exam Room.

4. What additional steps should have been taken by the medical assistant to make the patient more at ease about the procedure?

5. Why is it important for the patient to be in either a lying or sitting position during venipuncture?

6. True or False:

a. _____ Venipuncture may take place on the side of a mastectomy.

b. _____ Sclerosed veins feel hard and knotty and should not be used for venipuncture.

c. _____ Veins that are near the top of the skin are always the veins to use for venipuncture.

d. _____ The angle of the needle for venipuncture is 15 degrees.

e. _____ When blood is being drawn from the back of the hand, a butterfly needle or winged infusion set is more comfortable and more likely to provide a quality specimen.

f. _____ The tourniquet should be placed on the arm approximately 4 inches above the venipuncture site when finding the appropriate vein and should remain in place until after the venipuncture is complete, no matter how long the time.

g. _____ The tourniquet should remain in place until after the needle is removed following venipuncture.

 • Remain in the Exam Room with Kevin McKinzie and continue to Exercise 3.

Exercise 3

 Writing Activity—Disposal of Supplies and Handling of Specimen Following Venipuncture

 20 minutes

• Once again, we will continue with Mr. McKinzie's visit. (*Note:* If you have exited the program, sign in again to Mountain View Clinic, select Kevin McKinzie, and go to the Exam Room.)

1. After venipuncture, what is the proper procedure for disposal of the venipuncture supplies?

 • From the Exam Room menu, click on **Clean Room**.

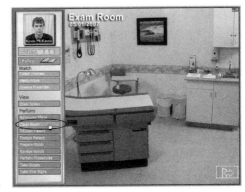

Click on Clean Room.

➡ • Select the appropriate steps to clean the Exam Room after Mr. McKinzie's visit; then click **Finish**.

• Click the exit arrow to return to the Summary Menu.

• Click on **Look at Your Performance Summary** and compare your answers with those of the experts. This summary can be saved or printed for your instructor.

• Click on **Close** and then on **Return to Map**.

2. True or False:

a. _____ OSHA has designated that safety-engineered devices on needles should be used to prevent needlestick injuries.

b. _____ After venipuncture, all materials that have come in contact with the skin must be disposed in biohazard waste.

c. _____ OSHA requires that hands be sanitized following venipuncture.

d. _____ The tourniquet used for the venipuncture should be sanitized using alcohol and may be used for another patient.

e. _____ Gloves may be removed immediately after the venipuncture, and the test tubes with no gross contamination may be handled without gloves.

f. _____ Handwashing/hand sanitization should be done after removing gloves and before documentation in the medical record.

g. _____ The length of time a specimen is held following venipuncture and before centrifuging has no significance.

h. _____ Specimens that are not handled with care may have hemolysis.

➡ • On the office map, click on **Laboratory** and then on **Charts**.

• Click on the **Diagnostic Tests** tab and select **1-Laboratory Requisition Form**.

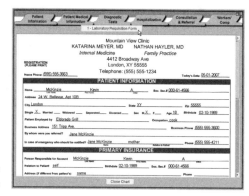

Under Diagnostic Tests,
select 1-Laboratory Requisition.

• Review the laboratory request to ensure that all tests that are not CLIA-waived have been ordered.

3. Did you find that the tests were correctly ordered?

4. Should any of the tests have been done on the next day because of the need to fast?

 • Click **Close Chart** to return to the Laboratory.
 • Now click on **Logs**.

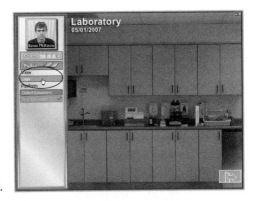

Click on Logs.

5. Are all of the tests properly logged for quality control and for following the results of the tests?

6. Use the blank log below to document the specimens for Kevin McKinzie as found in the physician's notes.

Requisition Number	Date of Specimen Collection	Patient Name	Laboratory Test	Processing Lab	Initials: Specimen Collection	Date of Results Return	Initials: Results Return

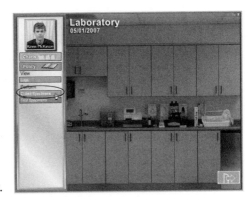 • Click on **Finish** to close the Log and return to the Laboratory.
 • Under Perform, click on **Test Specimens**.

Click on Test Specimens.

• A series of questions will be asked for each test selected. Answer all the questions related to each test and click **Finish** to return to the Laboratory. (*Hint:* The Policy Manual can be opened at any time for reference as you answer the questions.)

• Remain in the Laboratory with Kevin McKinzie and continue to Exercise 4.

Exercise 4

 CD-ROM Activity—Documentation of the Specimens

 5 minutes

• Let's continue with Mr. McKinzie's visit. (*Note:* If you have exited the program, sign in again to Mountain View Clinic, select Kevin McKinzie, and go to the Laboratory.)

• Click on **Charts** and then on **Diagnostic Tests**. From the drop-down menu, select **1-Laboratory Requisition Form** and review the tests performed on Mr. McKinzie.

1. Mr. McKinzie's appointment time was 2:45 p.m. Using this information and the tests ordered, document on the blank Progress Notes below the collection of the venipuncture specimens, including the laboratory to which the specimens were sent.

PATIENTS NAME	☐ FEMALE ☐ MALE	Date of Birth: / /
DATE	PATIENT VISITS AND FINDINGS	

ALLERGIC TO

ORDER #25-7193-01 · ©1999 BIBBERO SYSTEMS, INC. · PETALUMA, CA   TO REORDER CALL 800-BIBBERO (800-242-2376) OR FAX (800) 242-9330 MFG IN USA   PAGE ___ of ___

2. What information is lacking from the documentation of the venipuncture in the medical record?

3. What documentation should be placed on the tubes of blood before they are sent to the outside lab?

Exercise 5

Writing Activity—Performing Capillary Puncture on Infants and Older Children or Adults

 15 minutes

In this exercise you will determine the proper site for capillary puncture for infants and other patients by showing the proper sites on the drawings below. This information will be obtained from your textbook readings.

 1. On the figure below, show the proper sites for adult capillary puncture. (*Hint:* Refer to your textbook for this information.)

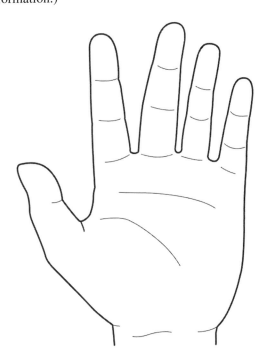

2. On the figure below, show the proper sites for infant capillary puncture. (*Hint:* Refer to your textbook for this information.)

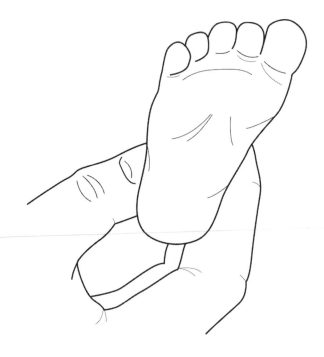

3. True or False:

a. _____ The site of puncture in an infant is important to prevent the possibility of nerve damage.

b. _____ The site of puncture in an older child or an adult is important to prevent the possibility of nerve damage.

c. _____ The proper selection of puncture site for an adult prevents unnecessary discomfort.

d. _____ The length of the lancet to be used for adults and infants is the same.

e. _____ The same collection containers used for venipuncture may be used for capillary punctures.

f. _____ Capillary puncture is used to obtain small amounts of blood, and the chance of infection is reduced by using this method because a larger blood vessel is not entered.

g. _____ Collection containers for capillary puncture have many of the same additives as those used for venipuncture.

h. _____ The plantar surface of the heel is used for infants who are not yet walking, but this is not the preferred site to use after a child begins walking.

i. _____ All fingers are acceptable sites for capillary puncture.

j. _____ Specimens obtained by capillary puncture should be handled as carefully as those from venipuncture to prevent hemolysis.

k. _____ Blood collected with a capillary puncture is pulled into the collection device either by capillary action or by being dropped onto a reagent strip for testing.

l. _____ Documentation of capillary puncture does not necessarily include the site of puncture, but this information should be included for infants.

m. _____ When specimens are collected by capillary puncture, the usual documentation needed for legal purposes is the type of test performed.

n. _____ The same safety precautions used with venipuncture should be used with capillary puncture.

o. _____ Because of the added chance of contamination of surfaces by blood, it is wise to have extra supplies such as gloves, gauze pads, and disinfectant readily available.

4. Capillary puncture is appropriate under which of the following conditions? Select all that apply.

_____ Only a small amount of blood needed for the sample

_____ A patient who is afraid of needles and prefers a capillary puncture to draw all specimens

_____ Older patients who have small rolling veins that are difficult to enter and for whom the test can be performed with a small amount of blood

_____ Pediatric patients who are not yet able to walk

_____ Patient who needs frequent blood samples such as a person with diabetes

_____ Teenagers who simply prefer the capillary puncture for all testing

_____ Persons who are obese, have scarring at venipuncture sites, have had mastectomies, or are at risk for venous thrombosis

Hematology

✐ **Reading Assignment:** Chapter 29—Introduction to the Clinical Laboratory
  • Blood Collection
  Chapter 32—Hematology

Patient: Louise Parlet

Objectives:

- Discuss what is meant by CLIA-waived laboratory testing.
- Discuss methods for obtaining specimens for CLIA-waived hematology testing.
- List the components of blood that are tested in a complete blood count.
- Discuss the difference between hemoglobin and hematocrit determinations and the normal range for each.
- List the normal ranges for RBC, WBC, and platelet counts.
- Describe the collection of a spun hematocrit.
- Discuss the difference in blood counts with polycythemia and leukemia.
- List the types of leukocytes.
- Discuss the need for quality control with hematology testing.
- Document lab test results on a laboratory flow sheet.

Exercise 1

  CD-ROM Activity—Performing Diagnostic Tests According to Office Policy

30 minutes

- Sign in to Mountain View Clinic.
- From the patient list, select **Louise Parlet**.

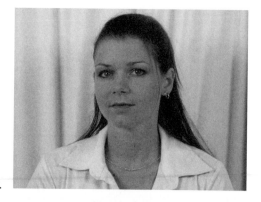

Select Louise Parlet.

- On the office map, highlight and click on **Exam Room** to enter the examination area.

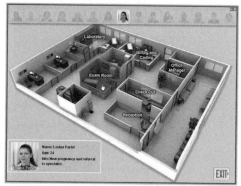

Click on Exam Room.

- Under the View heading, click on **Exam Notes** and read the initial documentation of Ms. Parlet's visit.

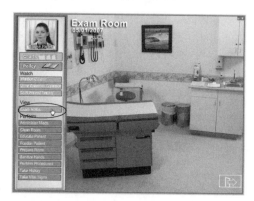

Click on Exam Notes.

- After reading the Exam Notes, click **Finish** to return to the Exam Room.
- Click on **Policy** to open the Policy Manual.

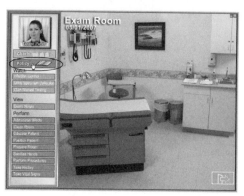

Click on Policy.

• In the search bar, type "standing orders" and click on the magnifying glass to read the section on standing orders, which ends on page 26 of the Policy Manual.

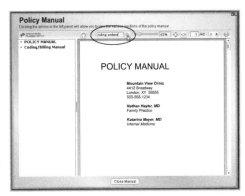

Type "standing orders" and click the magnifying glass.

• Leave the Policy Manual open to this page as you answer the following questions.

1. What is the primary diagnosis for Ms. Parlet?

2. According to office policy, what tests should be obtained from Ms. Parlet?

 • Return to the Policy Manual and read the section on Laboratory Policies that begins on page 27.

3. What is meant by CLIA?

4. The three levels of CLIA testing are:
   a. simple, moderate, and high complexity.
   b. waived, easy, and high complexity.
   c. waived, moderate, and high complexity.
   d. easy, medium, and complex complexity.
   e. waived, medium, and complex complexity.

5. Which of the following statements are true about CLIA-waived tests? Select all that apply.

   _____ CLIA-waived tests include those tests that could be performed by the patient.

   _____ CLIA-waived tests are of moderate complexity.

   _____ Laboratories performing only CLIA-waived tests do not need to register with HCFA.

_____ The CDC maintains a list of CLIA-waived tests.

_____ CLIA-waived tests are the most commonly performed lab tests.

_____ The most complex tests require personnel with special training for interpretation.

_____ The moderately complex CLIA testing requires specially trained laboratory personnel with special training for the tests performed.

_____ CLIA-waived tests include rapid strep testing, erythrocyte sedimentation rates, ovulation testing with visual color comparisons, and fecal occult blood testing.

_____ Microscopic analysis of urine is a CLIA-waived test.

_____ New methodologies for performing waived tests are added to the CDC website.

_____ CLIA testing requires quality control, quality assurance, and proficiency testing.

_____ Quality control involves testing equipment for efficiency.

_____ Quality assurance is the performance of tests to ensure the accuracy and reliability of the test results.

_____ Proficiency testing is a form of external quality control designed to ensure that the equipment and supplies being used are reliable and meet nationally accepted standards.

6. List at least four methods for obtaining CLIA-waived tests.

7. Which of the tests you identified in question 2 could be performed as CLIA-waived tests by the medical assistant before the physician sees the patient?

- Click **Close Manual** to return to the Exam Room.
- Click the exit arrow to go to the Summary Menu.
- Click **Return to Map**.
- On the office map, highlight and click on **Billing and Coding**.

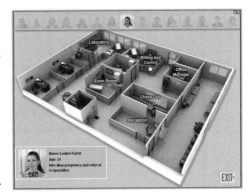

Click on Billing and Coding.

- Click on **Charts**.
- Next, click on the Patient Medical Information tab and select **3-Progress Notes** from the drop-down menu.

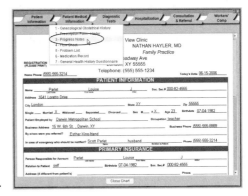

Select 3-Progress Notes.

- Read the final Progress Notes for Ms. Parlet's visit.
- Remain in Billing and Coding with Ms. Parlet to complete the remaining exercises.

8. According to the Progress Notes, what further blood tests were ordered for Ms. Parlet? Were any of these CLIA-waived?

Exercise 2

Writing Activity—Components of Hematology

  15 minutes

In this exercise, you will review hematology and its components.

1. Define *hematology*.

2. True or False:

a. _____ Many tests that previously were not CLIA-waived tests are now acceptable as CLIA-waived because of the advances in medical laboratory testing equipment.

b. _____ Hematology testing includes WBC, RBC, WBC differential, hemoglobin, hematocrit, ESR, platelet counts, and prothrombin times.

c. _____ A CBC (complete blood count) includes WBC, RBC, platelet count, Hgb, Hct, differential count, and RBC indices.

d. _____ Hemoglobin is a component of WBCs.

e. _____ Hemoglobin is the compound that allows the blood cells to transport oxygen.

f. _____ Leukocytes have the ability to phagocyte other cells.

g. _____ Thrombocytes are also called *platelets*.

h. _____ An abnormally high level of WBCs is often diagnosed as polycythemia.

i. _____ When a patient has high hemoglobin, it is often indicative of polycythemia.

j. _____ Leukocytosis may be a sign of leukemia.

k. _____ Hematocrit literally means "to separate blood."

l. _____ A CLIA-waived test to obtain hematocrit levels includes a spun hematocrit.

m. _____ A high hematocrit may indicate anemia.

n. _____ When capillary tubes are spun to obtain a spun hematocrit level, the two layers obtained are red blood cells and white blood cells.

o. _____ When a hematocrit sample is obtained from a capillary puncture, the first drop of blood should be discarded before collecting the sample.

3. Define *MCV*, *MCH*, and *MCHC*.

4. For each blood component listed below, identify the normal range for males and females.

Blood Component	Normal Range by Gender
Red blood cells (erythrocytes)	
White blood cells	
Hemoglobin (Hgb)	
Hematocrit (Hct)	
Platelets	
WBC differential	

5. Describe the collection of a capillary puncture specimen into a calibrated capillary tube for a spun hematocrit.

6. What should the medical assistant do if air bubbles are present in the capillary tube?

7. Why is it important for no air bubbles to be in the capillary puncture specimen for a spun hematocrit?

8. On the diagram below, label the cellular elements found in a capillary tube following centrifuging.

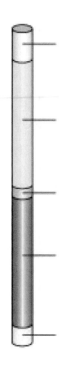

9. When a microhematocrit centrifuge is being used to spin a capillary tube, which of the following are necessary for safety? Select all that apply.

_____ Using PPEs

_____ Placing capillary tube anywhere in the centrifuge

_____ Placing capillary tubes opposite each other for balance

_____ Placing the sealed edge of the capillary tube toward the exterior of the centrifuge

_____ Placing the capillary tube toward the center of the centrifuge

_____ Closing the lid of the centrifuge before spinning the capillary tube

_____ Opening the lid immediately after the centrifuge stops the cycle

_____ Opening the lid when the centrifuge stops spinning

Exercise 3

Writing Activity—Documenting Hematology Testing

20 minutes

In this exercise you will document Louise Parlet's lab results in her Progress Notes and on the flow sheet.

1. The only CLIA-waived test documented for Ms. Parlet was her urine HCG. Her hemoglobin (Hgb), her glucose level, and a dipstick urine were also tested, but they were not documented until after the patient left the office at 9:45 a.m. On the blank Progress Notes below, document the following CLIA-waived test results for Ms. Parlet: Hgb 11.2; BS 115, NF; Dipstick urine Neg sugar, albumin, protein, leukocytes; pH 7; Sp gr 1.025.

PATIENT'S NAME	□ FEMALE □ MALE	Date of Birth: / /
DATE	PATIENT VISITS AND FINDINGS	

ALLERGIC TO

ORDER #25-7133-01 • © 1999 BIBBERO SYSTEMS, INC. • PETALUMA, CA   TO REORDER CALL 800-BIBBERO (800-242-2376) OR FAX (800) 242-9330 MFG IN USA   PAGE _____ of _____

2. Below is the first page of Ms. Parlet's flow sheet. Fill in the results from the CLIA-waived testing performed during her visit. (*Note:* Some results will be recorded in question 3.)

FLOW SHEET

Name: *Louise Parlet*   **Date of Birth**: *07/04/1982* **Age**:   23

Vital Signs	Date:	05/01/07									
Weight		125 lbs									
Height		5 ft 5 in									
Temperature		98.2 F									
Pulse		72									
Respirations		16									
Blood Pressure		104/72									
Lab Tests	Date:	05/01/07									
CBC											
RBC											
WBC											
HGB											
Hematocrit											
AlkalinePhosphatase											
Albumin											
Glucose											
Bilirubin total											
BUN											
Calcium											
Cholesterol											
Chloride											
CO2											
Creatinine											
Hb A1c											

3. Now complete page 2 of the flow sheet with the remaining CLIA-waived testing results.

LipidProfile										
LDL										
HDL										
Triglycerides										
SGGT										
SGOG/AST										
SGPT/ATL										
LDH										
T3										
T4										
T7										
TSH										
Triglycerides										
Total Protein										
Uric Acid										
Sodium										
Potassium										
Urinalysis										
Albumin										
Glucose										
PAPSmear										
PSA										
Other tests:										

4. Dr. Hayler received a partial report on Ms. Parlet's lab results today. Document the results in the blank Progress Notes below, using today's date and time and the following results: Hgb 10.6; Hct 38%; RBC 4.2; WBC 5400; Platelet count 200,000; Preg test Pos; Rubella titer 1:1 (assumed immune); ABO O+; Rh+; PAP Neg; Chlamydia Neg.

PATIENT'S NAME	☐ FEMALE ☐ MALE	Date of Birth: / /
DATE	PATIENT VISITS AND FINDINGS	

ALLERGIC TO _____

PAGE ____ of ____

ORDER #25-7133-01 · © 1999 BIBBERO SYSTEMS, INC. · PETALUMA, CA   TO REORDER CALL 800-BIBBERO (800-242-2376) OR FAX (800) 242-9330 MFG IN USA

5. Below, begin documenting the lab results from the Progress Notes onto the flow sheet. (*Note:* You will complete the documentation in question 6.)

FLOW SHEET

Name: *Louise Parlet*   **Date of Birth**: *07/04/1982* **Age**: *23*

Vital Signs	Date:	05/01/07								
Weight		125 lbs								
Height		5 ft 5 in								
Temperature		98.2 F								
Pulse		72								
Respirations		16								
Blood Pressure		104/72								
Lab Tests	**Date:**	05/01/07								
CBC										
RBC										
WBC										
HGB		11.2								
Hematocrit										
AlkalinePhosphatase										
Albumin										
Glucose		115 NF								
Bilirubin total										
BUN										
Calcium										
Cholesterol										
Chloride										
CO2										
Creatinine										
Hb A1c										

6. Now complete page 2 of the flow sheet with the remaining lab results.

LipidProfile										
LDL										
HDL										
Triglycerides										
SGGT										
SGOG/AST										
SGPT/ATL										
LDH										
T3										
T4										
T7										
TSH										
Triglycerides										
Total Protein										
Uric Acid										
Sodium										
Potassium										
Urinalysis										
Albumin	neg									
Glucose	neg									
PAPSmear										
PSA										
Other tests: *urine HcG*	pos									

7. Should any of Ms. Parlet's lab test results be highlighted for the physician for special attention? If so, which one(s)?

Blood Chemistry and Serology

Patient: Rhea Davison

Objectives:

- Describe the CLIA-waived chemistry tests commonly seen in a medical office.
- Discuss the necessity of quality control for blood glucose tests in home and office testing.
- Explain the purposes of chemistry testing.
- Identify the normal ranges of more commonly performed chemistry testing.
- Discuss the needed preparation for a fasting blood glucose test.
- Describe the difference between fasting chemistry testing and 2-hour postprandial chemistry testing.
- Indicate which tests should be obtained as fasting chemistry tests when possible.
- State the patient teaching important in obtaining blood glucose tests using an Accu-Chek glucose meter.
- Describe the proper storage of blood glucose testing supplies.
- Complete the laboratory log for specimens being sent to an outside lab.
- Document the test results on a laboratory flow sheet and indicate those tests that need to be seen by the physician as soon as possible.

Exercise 1

Writing Activity—Common Blood Chemistry Testing

20 minutes

1. What is measured through blood chemistry testing?

2. What is the most common type of specimen collected for a blood chemistry? Why is this the type of specimen needed?

3. Name three blood chemistry tests that are commonly performed in the medical office laboratory.

4. What preparation is needed for most blood chemistry testing in the medical office?

5. What is the best appointment time for the patient to have a blood chemistry test?

6. Give the normal ranges for the following blood chemistry components.

   a. BUN:

   b. Fasting blood glucose:

   c. 2-hour PPBS:

   d. Total cholesterol:

   e. LDL cholesterol:

   f. HDL cholesterol:

   g. Triglycerides:

7. What are some side effects that may occur in a patient who is having a glucose tolerance test?

Exercise 2

 CD-ROM Activity—Patient Education for Quality Blood Glucose Tests

 30 minutes

- Sign in to Mountain View Clinic.
- From the patient list, select **Rhea Davison**.

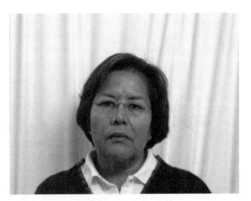

Rhea Davison

- On the office map, highlight and click on **Exam Room**.

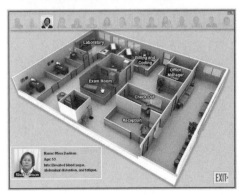

Click on Exam Room.

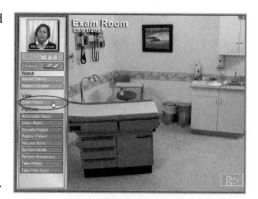

➤ • In the Exam Room, click on **Exam Notes** to read the initial documentation of Ms. Davison's visit.

Click on Exam Notes.

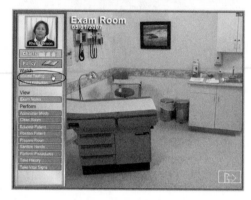

• Close the notes to return to the Exam Room.
• Under the Watch heading, click on **Waived Testing** to view the video.
• Click **Close** at the end of the video to return to the Exam Room.

Click on Waived Testing.

1. Now that you have read the Exam Notes and watched the video, why do you think that Dr. Meyer wants Ms. Davison to perform a glucose test using the equipment in the office?

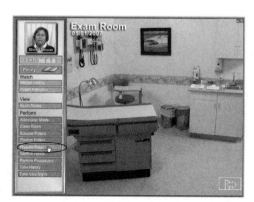

➤ • Remain in the Exam Room with Ms. Davison and select **Prepare Room** from the Perform menu.

Select Prepare Room.

LESSON 24—BLOOD CHEMISTRY AND SEROLOGY   255

 • Select the first item needed for Ms. Davison's visit from the alphabetical list and click **Add Item** to confirm your choice. Each item you add will appear in the Selected Supplies box.

• Repeat this step until you are satisfied you have everything you need from the list. Leave this window open as you answer the following questions. (*Reminder:* The Exam Notes are available if you need to refer to them.)

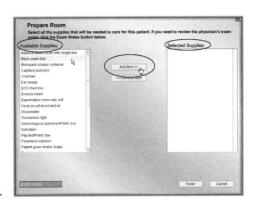

Select the necessary supplies.

2. List the supplies needed by a medical assistant for blood glucose testing.

3. Which of the following supplies would be needed by Ms. Davison for performing quality control of the glucose testing equipment she currently uses at home? Select all that apply.

_____ Abnormal control sample

_____ Gloves

_____ Normal control

_____ Glucose meter

_____ Sterile wipes

_____ Container for sharps

_____ Glucose reagent strips

_____ Capillary lancet

 • Click **Finish** to return to the Exam Room.

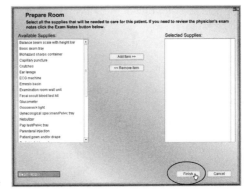

Click Finish.

Copyright © 2009 by Saunders, an imprint of Elsevier Inc. All rights reserved.

4. True or False:

    a. _____ All chemistry tests results are confined to only a single number for normal readings.

    b. _____ Cholesterol and blood glucose may be CLIA-waived tests.

    c. _____ To perform cholesterol and blood glucose testing in the medical office, the equipment must be CLIA-waived unless highly qualified personnel are available for the testing.

    d. _____ At home, a patient should store equipment away from light and heat sources.

    e. _____ Blood chemistry testing may give qualitative results.

    f. _____ Blood chemistry testing may give quantitative results.

    g. _____ Blood chemistry testing is used for differential diagnoses.

    h. _____ The equipment used by patients at home is CLIA-waived.

    i. _____ All types of blood glucose equipment have the same instructions for use.

5. What information needs to be supplied to Ms. Davison about the collection of the specimen immediately following the capillary puncture?

6. What information should be supplied to Ms. Davison about the use of the glucose meter?

7. The medical assistant suggests that Ms. Davison ask the physician for a new glucose testing meter. Why do you think this is important?

8. In the Exam Notes, Ms. Davison reports having missed several doses of medication because of the inability to buy the medication. How would you expect this to affect the test results she obtained at home?

9. Would you expect Ms. Davison to have an increase in weight if she is following her pre-scribed diet? Explain your answer.

 • Click the exit arrow to leave the Exam Room.
• To continue with this lesson, click on **Return to Map**. (*Note:* If you wish to see your Prepare Room exercise results, first click on **Look at Your Performance Summary** and compare your answers against the experts.)

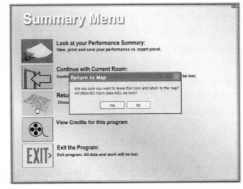

Click on Return to Map.

• On the office map highlight and click on **Check Out** to review the final documentation of Rhea Davison's visit.

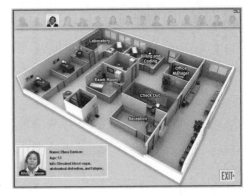

Click on Check Out.

• Click on **Charts** and select **1-Progress Notes** from the drop-down menu under the **Patient Medical Information** tab.

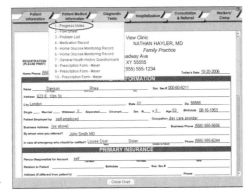

Select 1-Progress Notes.

• Read the results of today's blood glucose test and the testing that is to be done on the next day.
• Remain at the Check Out desk with Ms. Davison's Progress Notes available to answer the remaining questions in this exercise.

10. Is the test result for Ms. Davison's blood glucose obtained in the office within the limits expected when compared with the results from her home testing? Explain your answer.

11. Dr. Meyer ordered an HgbA1c. What information does this test provide? Why is this an important test for Dr. Meyer to use in treating Ms. Davison?

Exercise 3

Writing Activity—Quality Control with Blood Chemistry Testing

15 minutes

In this exercise you will use your knowledge to decide whether quality control has been accomplished.

1. True or False:

   a. _____ Quality control for blood chemistry testing should be done no more than once a day.

   b. _____ When new reagent strips are opened, quality control sampling should occur.

   c. _____ Quality control samples have expiration dates.

   d. _____ Quality control samples may be used with any equipment.

   e. _____ Quality control is performed only so that the physician will have an accurate reading for comparison.

   f. _____ If the quality control samples are consistently inaccurate, the patient should try to repair the equipment used at home, because the patient is the person who best understands how that specific equipment works.

   g. _____ One method of checking for quality control of a machine in the medical office is to compare results obtained from a reference lab on a specific specimen with the results obtained on that same specimen in the office laboratory.

2. What is the significance if samples for quality control fall out of the control range?

3. If a patient questions the importance of performing quality control on a regular basis, what should you tell the patient?

Exercise 4

 CD-ROM Activity—Preparing a Laboratory Log for Patient Specimens

 15 minutes

1. Rhea Davison's specimens were sent to an outside lab (Quality Lab) the day following her appointment. Using her Progress Notes, prepare the laboratory log below for these tests. (*Note:* The requisition number has been filled in for you.)

Requisition Number	Date of Specimen Collection	Patient Name	Laboratory Test	Processing Lab	Initials: Specimen Collection	Date of Results Return	Initials: Results Return
112417							

Exercise 5

 CD-ROM Activity—Adding Laboratory Results to the Flow Sheet

 15 minutes

1. Using the flow sheet pages below and in question 2 on the next page, transfer the test results recorded in Ms. Davison's Progress Notes for 5-1-07. Also add the following results, which were received by Dr. Meyer on 5-3-07. Place an asterisk (*) after any results that should be given prompt attention.

Additional results from 5-3-07:

- Blood chemistry: Albumin 4.2; Alk phos 4; Bilirubin 1.2; SCOT 14; Bicarbonate 21; Calcium 7.2; Chloride 98; Creatinine 0.6; LDH 96; Glucose 460; Potassium 4.8; Total protein 6.6; Sodium 130; Urea nitrogen 18; Phosphorus 3.2
- Thyroid profile: T4 10.8; T3 185; TSH 15.4
- CA 125: 3.6
- HgbA1c: 10

FLOW SHEET

Name: Rhea Davison   Date of Birth: 08/16/1953   Age: 53

Vital Signs	Date:	05/01/07								
Weight		152								
Height		5 ft 1 in								
Temperature		98.6								
Pulse		86								
Respirations		24								
Blood Pressure		144/86								
Lab Tests	**Date:**									
CBC										
RBC										
WBC										
HGB										
Hematocrit										
AlkalinePhosphatase										
Albumin										
Glucose										
Bilirubin total										
BUN										
Calcium										
Cholesterol										
Chloride										
CO2										
Creatinine										
Hb A1c										

2. Below, continue documenting Ms. Davison's lab results on the second page of the flow sheet. (*Reminder:* Use the data from her Progress Notes on 5-1-07 and the additional results received by Dr. Meyer on 5-3-07, listed in question 1. Place an asterisk (*) after any results that should be given prompt attention.)

LipidProfile										
LDL										
HDL										
Triglycerides										
SGGT										
SGOG/AST										
SGPT/ATL										
LDH										
T3										
T4										
T7										
TSH										
Triglycerides										
Total Protein										
Uric Acid										
Sodium										
Potassium										
Urinalysis										
Albumin										
Glucose										
PAPSmear										
PSA										
Other tests:										

Medical Microbiology

⌀ **Reading Assignment:** Chapter 34—Medical Microbiology

Patient: Tristan Tsosie

Objectives:

- Discuss the difference between pathogens and nonpathogens.
- Describe the proper procedure for obtaining microbiological specimens for testing.
- Identify the correct handling and transportation of a microbiological specimen.
- Discuss the need to use standard precautions when obtaining microbiological specimens.
- Demonstrate the correct documentation of microbiological specimen collection.

Exercise 1

 CD-ROM Activity—Obtaining a Wound Specimen for Microbiological Testing

30 minutes

- Sign in to Mountain View Clinic.
- From the patient list, select **Tristan Tsosie**.

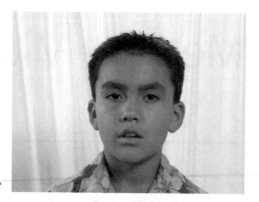

Tristan Tsosie

- On the office map, click to enter the **Exam Room**.

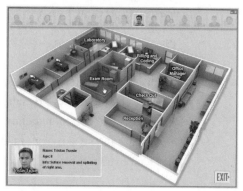

Click on Exam Room.

- From the Exam Room menu, select **Wound Care** and watch the video.

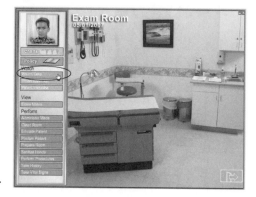

Click on Wound Care.

1. In the video, the medical assistant states that a wound specimen will be obtained for testing. Why is the wound specimen being taken from Tristan's arm?

2. Why should the specimen be taken before cleansing the wound?

• Click **Close** at the end of the video and return to the Exam Room.

• Next, click on **Exam Notes** to review the initial documentation of Tristan's visit.

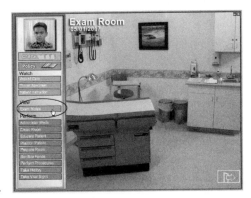

Click on Exam Notes.

3. What tests have been ordered for Tristan?

 • Click **Finish** to close the Exam Notes.

• Now select **Prepare Room** and choose the supplies and equipment needed for Tristan's exam. (*Note:* You can reopen the Exam Notes for reference as you make your selections.)

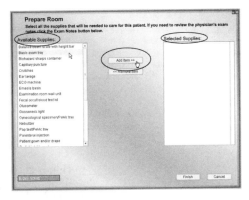

Select the supplies needed for this visit.

• After completing your selections, click **Finish** to return to the Exam Room.

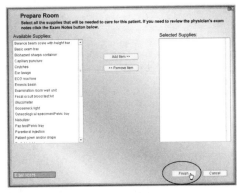

Click Finish to return to the Exam Room.

4. Describe the difference between pathogens and nonpathogens. Explain the importance of this in regard to wound care.

5. True or False:

a. _____ The wound specimen should be taken from the cleanest area of the wound.

b. _____ Wound specimens should be placed in the transport medium immediately after they are obtained.

c. _____ Wound specimens should be dry for transport so that the chance of cross contamination is reduced.

d. _____ Ideally, wound specimens should be obtained after antibiotic therapy has been initiated.

e. _____ Hands should be sanitized before and after collecting the specimen, even though gloves have been worn.

f. _____ Supplies used in the collection of the wound specimen should be disposed in the biohazardous waste.

g. _____ Collection of all wound specimens requires the use of gowns and goggles.

h. _____ Collection of the wound specimen is not complete until documentation has been completed.

i. _____ The time between collection of the specimen and the laboratory processing of the specimen is not important.

6. Describe the means used by the medical assistant and the extern to place Tristan at ease during the procedure of collecting the wound specimen.

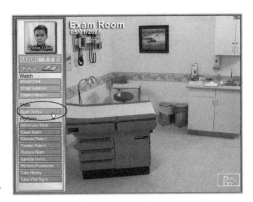

• From the Exam Room menu, again click on **Exam Notes** to read the documentation concerning the wound.

Click on Exam Notes.

7. Below are the Progress Notes from Tristan's chart, showing how the wound specimen collection was documented. Compare this documentation against the Exam Notes. Is there any information that could be, or should be, added to this documentation?

| 05-01-2007 11:45am | Wound culture obtained, wound cleaned, 7 stitches removed, and new posterior splint reapplied without apparent intolerance. Appears comfortable, no complaints. Fingers pink and warm. QuickVue In-Line One Step Strep A test done; results negative. Wound culture to be sent to QualityLab on 05/02/2007. Given verbal and written instructions on observing for signs of infection, proper splint care, and activity during the healing process. Instructed to have parent call in 2 days with update and to confirm understanding of follow-up care.-- ———————————————————————————*Cathy Wright, CMA* |
| 05-01-2007 12:00pm | Mother contacted and given instructions about required follow-up care.————————— ———————————————————————————*Leah Tran, CMA* |

• Click **Finish**, remain in the Exam Room with Tristan, and continue to Exercise 2.

Exercise 2

 CD-ROM Activity—Collecting a Throat Specimen for Microbiological Testing

 20 minutes

The Policy Manual does not specify the needed protective equipment for a professional who is obtaining a throat specimen but simply states that OSHA standard precautions should be followed.

1. What protective equipment should be worn by the medical assistant while obtaining a routine throat specimen? When is it necessary to include other PPEs, and what should these be?

• From the Exam Room menu, select **Throat Specimen** and watch the video.

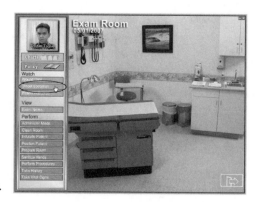

Click on Throat Specimen.

2. What did the medical assistant do to be sure that she had Tristan's cooperation?

 • Click the exit arrow to leave the Exam Room.
• On the Summary Menu, click on **Look at Your Performance Summary** to compare your answers with the experts.

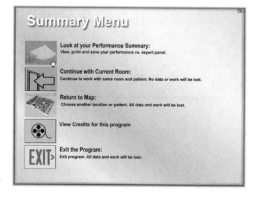

Click on Look at Your Performance Summary.

• Click on **Return to Map**.

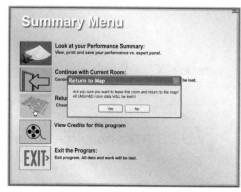

Click on Return to Map.

• On the office map, click to enter the
  Laboratory.

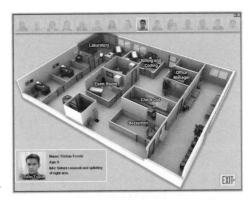

Click on Laboratory.

• Under Perform, select **Collect Specimens**.

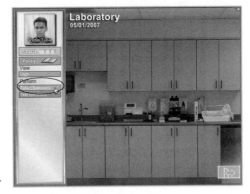

Click on Collect Specimens.

• Next, select all tests ordered for Tristan at this
  visit. (*Hint:* If you wish to review the notes for
  the visit, click on **Charts** and select **1-Progress
  Notes** under **Patient Medical Information**.)

• A series of questions will be asked for *each* test
  selected. Answer all questions related to each
  test and click **Finish** to return to the Laboratory.
  (*Hint:* The Policy Manual can be opened at any
  time for reference as you answer the questions.)

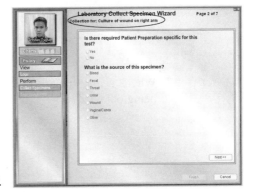

Answer the questions for each selected test.

• Open Tristan's chart (click on **Charts**) and select **1-Progress Notes** from the drop-down
  menu under the **Patient Medical Information** tab. Review as needed to answer the following
  questions.

3. What are the results of the strep test that was processed using the specimen?

4. Was the documentation correct for the testing done? Explain your answer.

5. When you are obtaining a throat specimen for testing, what is the most appropriate site for collection?

6. Why would it be advantageous to use two sterile swabs when collecting a specimen? In what situation(s) do you think a specimen would likely be sent to an outside lab?

7. Why is it important that the inside of the mouth not be touched while the throat specimen is being obtained?

➡ • Still in Tristan's chart, click on the **Diagnostic Tests** tab.
  • Select **3-Laboratory Requisition Form**.
  • Review the Laboratory Requisition Form for accuracy and completeness.

8. Is the Laboratory Requisition Form complete and correct? If not, describe any errors and explain what would need to be done to correct them.

9. What insurance information is to be provided with the requisition?

 • Click **Close Chart** to return to the Laboratory.
 • Under View, click on **Logs**.

10. Are all of the tests properly logged for quality control and for following the results of the tests?

11. On the blank log below, document the transport of the wound specimen to the lab.

Requisition Number	Date of Specimen Collection	Patient Name	Laboratory Test	Processing Lab	Initials: Specimen Collection	Date of Results Return	Initials: Results Return

 • Click **Finish** to return to the Exam Room.
 • Click the exit arrow and from the Summary Menu select **Look at Your Performance Summary**.
 • Expert responses are given separately for each test. Scroll down to locate the test you want to review. Your summary can also be printed or saved for your instructor.
 • Click **Close** and select **Return to Map**.

26

The Medical Record

Reading Assignment: Chapter 36—The Medical Record

Patients: Renee Anderson, Tristan Tsosie

Objectives:

- Discuss why proper organization of the medical record is essential.
- Identify and describe the forms found in a medical record.
- Apply principles of medical record organization to preparing a new patient's medical record.
- Select the forms that need to be added to the medical record for an established patient.
- Describe the appropriate care of a damaged medical record.
- Determine the appropriate division of medical records when a new record must be established.

Exercise 1

 CD-ROM Activity—Organizing a Medical Record for a New Patient

 30 minutes

- Sign in to Mountain View Clinic.
- From the patient list, select **Renee Anderson**.

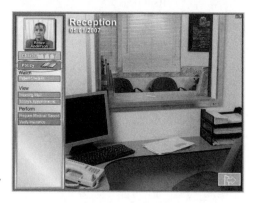

Renee Anderson

- Highlight and click on **Reception** on the office map.

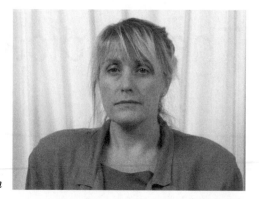

Click on Reception.

- Click on **Policy** to open the Policy Manual. In the search bar, type "medical record" and click on the magnifying glass to search.

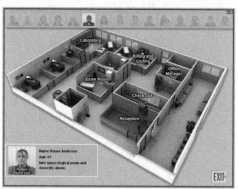

Click on Policy.
Then search for "medical record."

- Scroll up and down to read the duties assigned to the various types of medical assistants in the office.

1. At Mountain View Clinic, the Policy Manual states that the _____ medical assistant is responsible for preparing and organizing the medical record.

2. Why is it important for the administrative medical assistant to provide the necessary forms in a medical record for a new patient?

• When you have finished reading the relevant policy, click on **Close Manual** to return to the Reception desk.

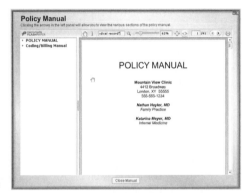

Click on Close Manual.

• At the Reception desk, click on **Prepare Medical Record** (under the Perform heading) to begin assembling a chart for Ms. Anderson's visit.

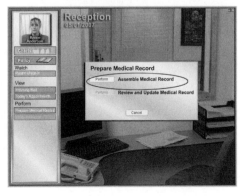

Click on Prepare Medical Record.

• Next to Assemble Medical Record, click on **Perform** to begin selecting the forms necessary for Ms. Anderson's visit.

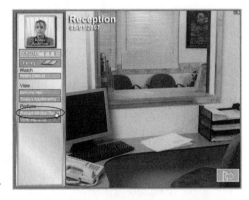

Click on Perform
(next to Assemble Medical Record).

- The Patient Information tab is automatically chosen as the starting point when you access the Assemble Medical Record screen. Under Forms Available, choose the forms that should be filed under the Patient Information tab. Click **Add** to complete your selections. (*Note:* To select multiple consecutive forms, hold down the Shift key while making your selections. To make multiple nonconsecutive selections, hold down the Control [Ctrl] key as you click on your choices.)

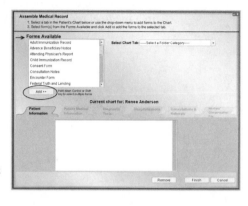

Make selections from Forms Available and click Add.

- When you have completed the Patient Information section, continue adding forms to the appropriate tabs in Renee Anderson's medical record. To select a new tab, either click on the tab on the medical record itself or use the drop-down menu to the right of Select Chart Tab.

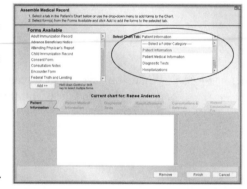

Select a chart tab to assemble.

- If you change you mind about a form you have added to a tab, click to highlight the name of the form and then click on **Remove** at the bottom of the screen.

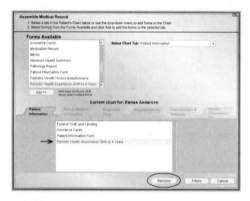

Click Remove to delete a form.

- When you are satisfied that you have selected all the necessary forms and put them in the correct tab sections, click **Finish** to close the medical record.

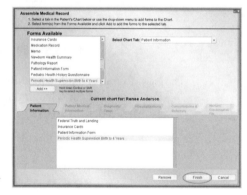

Click Finish.

• Now click on the exit arrow at the bottom of screen to leave the Reception area.
• On the Summary Menu, click on **Look at Your Performance Summary** to compare your answers against those of the experts. How did you do?

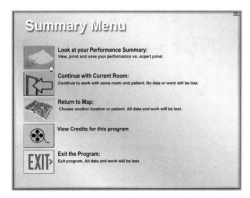

Click on Look at Your Performance Summary.

• The icons for saving and printing the Performance Summary are located at the top right corner of the screen.

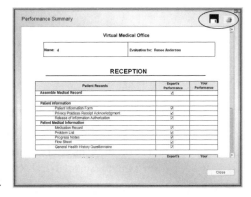

Save and/or print your summary.

• Click **Close**.
• Click **Return to Map**. (*Note:* If you did not save your Performance Summary, all data will be lost when you return to the map.)

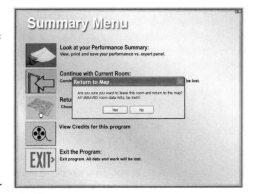

Click on Return to Map.

3. The form that contains the patient's demographic information is the

_____.

4. The form in the medical record that contains subjective information about the patient's

illnesses in the past is the _____.

5. The legal document that must be signed to allow information to be used to file insurance is

the _____.

6. The form that allows the physician to record findings in the medical record is the

_____.

Exercise 2

 CD-ROM Activity—Adding to the Medical Record of an Established Patient

 20 minutes

- From the patient list, click on **Tristan Tsosie**. (*Note:* If you have exited the program, sign in again to Mountain View Clinic and select Trsitan Tsosie from the patient list.)

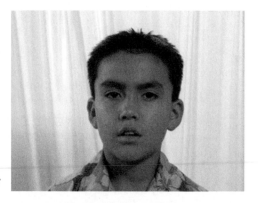

Tristan Tsosie

- On the office map, click on **Reception**.
- At the Reception desk, click on **Charts**.
- Click on the **Hospitalization** tab. From the drop-down menu, select **1-ED Record**.

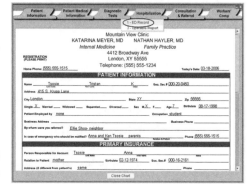

Click on Hospitalization; then click on 1-ED Record.

- Read the ED Record to decide what other forms should be available for the physician for this office visit and to determine whether Tristan is following the orders of the physician who saw him in the Emergency Department.
- Click on **Close Chart** to return to the Reception area.
- Under the Perform heading, select **Prepare Medical Record**.
- Click on the **Perform** button next to Review and Update Medical Records.

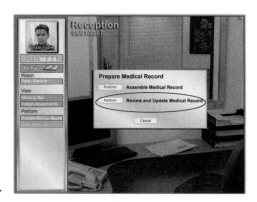

Review and Update Medical Records.

• Check the forms in each chart tab to be sure that the needed information for this visit is located under the correct tab and will be available when the physician needs it. Add any forms that you think are needed for this visit. If you think it is necessary, you may also remove or move any forms within the chart. (*Note:* If you need help with these steps, see the detailed instructions in Exercise 1 of this lesson.)

• Click **Finish** when you are done.

1. Was Tristan's follow-up appointment made at the appropriate time as directed by the physician in the Emergency Department?

2. What report(s), other than the ED Record, should have been added to the medical record for it to be complete for the physician?

3. When adding a form to the medical record, the medical assistant should:
   a. be sure the physician has seen the report before filing it.
   b. place the forms in the medical record in chronological order, with the earliest record on top.
   c. always be sure the date of arrival has been stamped on the form.
   d. wait to file the form just before the patient's arrival for an appointment.
   e. do both *a* and *d*.

4. When the medical assistant files materials in the medical record of an established patient, the materials should be filed in what order?

5. When accessing Tristan's medical record on arrival, you notice that the forms from the hospital have been torn during transmittal. What steps do you need to take to maintain the record from further damage?

6. If a patient's folder is old, torn, or simply worn, what should the medical assistant do?

7. Let's assume that a chart is overcrowded and a second chart needs to be established. In moving records to the new chart, how far back should those records go that are moved to the new chart? How should the record be marked to show that more than one medical record is available?

LESSON 27

Health History

Reading Assignment: Chapter 36—The Medical Record

Patients: Kevin McKinzie, Hu Huang, Tristan Tsosie, Wilson Metcalf

Objectives:

- State the need for a health history.
- Describe the components of the health history and the importance of each.
- State the questions that should be included during a health history.
- Indicate the accurate method of documenting a health history in a medical record.
- Demonstrate accurate written communication skills.
- Describe the correct documentation of the health history in the Progress Notes.
- Explain the difference between signs and symptoms.
- Differentiate between objective and subjective symptoms.
- Explain the need for confidentiality when obtaining a health history.

Exercise 1

Writing Activity—Background for Obtaining a Health History

30 minutes

1. What components should be included when you obtain a health history?

2. When obtaining a patient's past medical history, why is it important that the medical assistant review this information with the patient rather than just rely on what the patient writes on the form?

3. Why would the physician need to know any previous surgical procedures a patient has undergone and where these procedures were done?

4. What is included in a social history?

5. Why is it important to include educational background in a medical history?

6. Why are environmental factors important to include in a medical history?

7. Define *chief complaint*.

8. What four questions should the patient be asked to obtain an accurate chief complaint for documentation?

9. An expansion of the chief complaint occurs in the section of the health history called the

_____.

10. True or False:

    a. _____ The chief complaint should be exact and written in as many words as needed to convey the idea.

    b. _____ The chief complaint should be kept concise, with any additional information saved for the present illness history.

    c. _____ If possible, the chief complaint should be documented in the patient's own words.

    d. _____ The medical assistant should use accurate medical terminology when documenting the chief complaint.

    e. _____ The medical assistant may use diagnostic terminology when documenting the chief complaint.

    f. _____ The medical assistant should identify diseases in documenting the chief complaint.

    g. _____ It is important to obtain as complete a family history as possible to help with early diagnoses of familial diseases.

    h. _____ Familial diseases are those that affect blood relatives.

    i. _____ Documentation should be clear, concise, and correct.

j. _____ It is acceptable to write over a mistake when you are documenting.

k. _____ Any mistakes made during documentation should be dated and signed.

l. _____ Documentation should occur immediately after a procedure is performed.

m. _____ All documentation should be signed by the person who performed the task.

n. _____ When you are documenting, it is acceptable to use abbreviations that are common in your local area, even if these are not those commonly seen in the medical office.

11. Subjective symptoms are sometimes simply called _____, whereas

objective symptoms are called _____.

12. How are subjective symptoms obtained?

13. How are objective symptoms obtained?

14. Why is it important that the medical assistant ask questions of the patient in a private area rather than in the reception area?

Exercise 2

 CD-ROM Activity—Obtaining a Medical History from a New Patient

 30 minutes

- Sign in to Mountain View Clinic.
- From the patient list, select **Kevin McKinzie**.

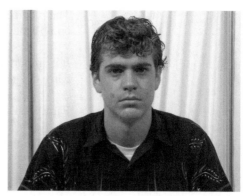

Kevin McKinzie

• On the office map, highlight and click on **Reception**.

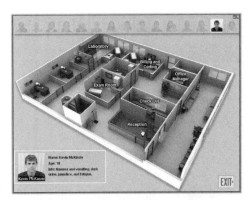

Click on Reception.

• Under the Watch heading, select **Patient Check-In** to view the video.

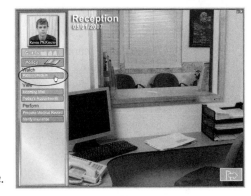

Click on Patient Check-In.

• Click **Close** at the end of the video to return to Reception.

1. Kevin McKinzie brings a history form to the medical office with him. What are the disadvantages of having the patient complete the medical history at home?

2. The administrative medical assistant takes the medical history and places it in a chart without reviewing it for completeness. Is this good practice? Explain your answer.

3. Would you have handled the check-in of Mr. McKinzie differently? If yes, explain how. Did the medical assistant respond adequately to the patient's verbal and nonverbal communication?

 • Click the exit arrow at the bottom right of the screen to leave the Reception area.

• On the Summary Menu, click **Return to Map**.

• On the office map, highlight and click on **Exam Room** to continue with Mr. McKinzie's visit.

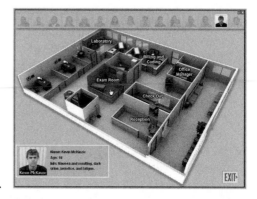

Click on Exam Room.

• From the menu on the left, click on **Charts** and select **1-General Health History Questionnaire** from the drop-down menu under the **Patient Medical Information** tab.

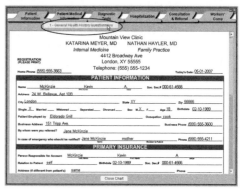

Click on 1-General Health History Questionnaire.

• Using the arrow at the top right of the questionnaire, turn to page 2.

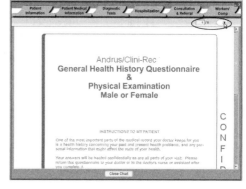

Open page 2.

• Thoroughly review the information Mr. McKinzie provided on page 2 of the questionnaire.

4. What is the patient's chief complaint as documented under Current Medical History?

5. What are two areas of Mr. McKinzie's social history that could have a bearing on this illness?

→ • Again using the arrow at the top of the screen, turn to page 3 of the questionnaire.
   • Thoroughly review the information Mr. McKinzie provided regarding his past history.

6. What, if any, familial history is relevant to his chief complaint?

→ • Still in the chart, click on the **Patient Information** tab and select **1-Patient Information Form**.

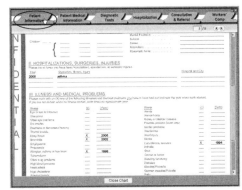

Click on Patient Information; then select 1-Patient Information Form.

• Read the Patient Information Form to find Mr. McKinzie's type of employment.
• Click **Close Chart** to return to the Exam Room.
• Click on **Exam Notes** (under View) and read the clinical diagnoses as documented by Dr. Hayler.

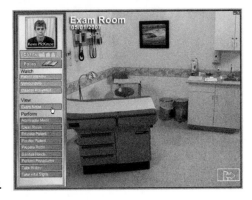

Click on Exam Notes.

• Click **Finish** to close the Exam Notes and return to the Exam Room.

7. What are the indications for patient education and infection control for these clinical diagnoses?

- Click the exit arrow to leave the Exam Room.
- On the Summary Menu, click **Return to Map** and continue to the next exercise.

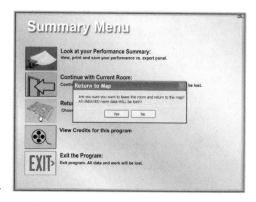

Click on Return to Map.

Exercise 3

 CD-ROM Activity—Documentation of Chief Complaint for Established Patient

 30 minutes

- From the patient list, select **Hu Huang**. (*Note:* If you have exited the program, sign in again to Mountain View Clinic and select Hu Huang from the patient list.)

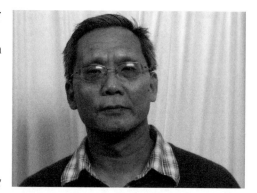

Hu Huang

- On the office map, highlight and click on **Exam Room**.
- Under the Watch heading, select **Respiratory Care** to view the video.

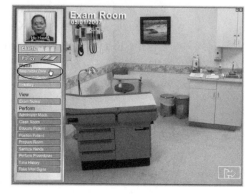

Click on Respiratory Care.

- Click **Close** at the end of the video to return to the Exam Room.
- Click on **Exam Notes** (under View) to read the documentation of Mr. Huang's visit.

1. What is your assessment of the verbal and nonverbal communication that Charlie conducted with Mr. Huang in the video?

2. What is the chief complaint for Mr. Huang?

3. Which of the symptoms listed are subjective symptoms?

4. What are the objective symptoms?

5. What other information could be placed in the History section of the Progress Notes?

6. Why was it important to obtain the information that Mr. Huang had been in China for several months?

➤ • Click **Finish** to close the Exam Notes and return to the Exam Room.
   • Open Mr. Huang's **Chart** and select **1-Progress Notes** from the drop-down menu under the **Patient Medical Information** tab.

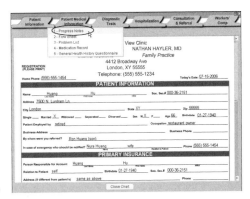

Select 1-Progress Notes.

• Read the documentation from all of Mr. Huang's previous visits.

7. After reading the Progress Notes for all his visits, what questions would have been appropriate for the medical assistant to ask Mr. Huang regarding medication compliance?

8. True or False:

a. _____ The chief complaint for an established patient should be documented in Progress Notes unless a new history/physical exam form is being completed.

b. _____ When documenting the chief complaint in the medical record of an established patient, the same questions of when, where, how, and how long should be asked.

c. _____ After the physician identifies a diagnosis, it is permissible for the medical assistant to use that diagnosis in documentation of the chief complaint.

d. _____ Proper spelling is not as important when documenting the care of an established patient since the physician has already spelled the medical terminology correctly in earlier Progress Notes.

e. _____ Documentation for an established patient is just as important as for a new patient.

f. _____ If the medical office has specific guidelines concerning documentation, these are not as important as those taught in class and should not be followed.

g. _____ When documenting in any medical record, the extern or medical assisting student should sign the medical record with the indication of student medical assistant (SMA).

h. _____ The medical assistant should document both objective and subjective symptoms in the medical record.

i. _____ If the physician has used a local abbreviation in the medical record, it is acceptable for the medical assistant to also use this abbreviation.

j. _____ Only clinical medical assistants document in medical records.

➤ • Click **Close Chart** to return to the Exam Room.
  • Click the exit arrow to leave the Exam Room.
  • Select **Return to Map** from the Summary Menu.

Exercise 4

  CD-ROM Activity—Documentation by Administrative Medical Assistants

15 minutes

- From the patient list, select **Tristan Tsosie**. (*Note:* If you have exited the program, sign in again to Mountain View Clinic and select Tristan Tsosie from the patient list.)

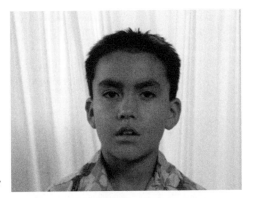

Tristan Tsosie

- On the office map, highlight and click on **Reception** to enter the check-in area.
- Under the Watch heading, click on **Patient Check-In** to view the video.

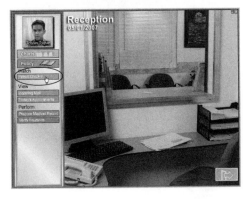

Click on Patient Check-In.

1. What important subjective symptoms does Tristan's sister report to the administrative medical assistant?

- Click the exit arrow to leave the Reception desk.
- Select **Return to Map** from the Summary Menu.
- Keeping Tristan as your patient, highlight and click on **Check Out** on the office map.

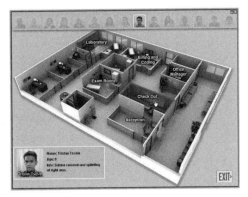

Click on Check Out.

- Next, click **Charts** and select **1-Progress Notes** from under the **Patient Medical Information** tab.
- Read the initial documentation written by Dana Brick, CMA.

2. Which of the four questions that should be asked for accurate documentation of chief complaint has been omitted from the Progress Notes, even though the sister provided the needed information when Tristan checked in?

3. Dana is a clinical medical assistant, and Kristin is an administrative medical assistant. Did the correct medical assistant document the information from the sister in the medical record?

4. How did you feel about the verbal and nonverbal communication between Kristin and Tristan and his sister during check-in? If you think there was a problem, how could it have been better handled?

  • Click **Close Chart**; then click on the exit arrow.
  • Select **Return to Map** from the Summary Menu and continue to the next exercise.

Exercise 5

Writing Activity—Practicing Documentation of History and Chief Complaint

45 minutes

  • From the patient list, select **Wilson Metcalf**. (*Note:* If you have exited the program, sign in again to Mountain View Clinic and select Wilson Metcalf from the patient list.)

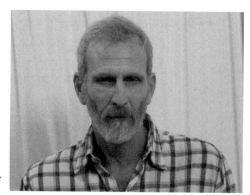

Wilson Metcalf

• On the office map, highlight and click on **Check Out**.

- Click on **Charts** and then select **1-Progress Notes** from the drop-down menu under the **Patient Medical Information** tab.

- Read the Progress Notes for Wilson Metcalf beginning with his initial visit to the office on 1-4-2007.

1. According to the Progress Notes, what were Mr. Metcalf's drinking habits at the time of his visit on 1-4-07?

2. How much coffee did Mr. Metcalf admit to drinking in a day?

 • Scroll down in the Progress Notes and read the documentation for the chief complaint for Mr. Metcalf's visit on 5-1-2007.

3. What are Mr. Metcalf's drinking habits now?

4. How much coffee does he admit to drinking at this visit?

5. What was the diagnosis documented by Dr. Meyer on 1-4-2007?

6. What is Mr. Metcalf's diagnosis on 5-1-2007?

→ • Click on the **Patient Medical Information** tab again; this time, select **5-General Health History Questionnaire**.

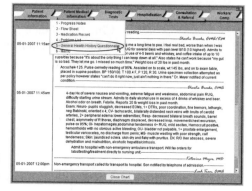

Click on 5-General Health History Questionnaire.

• Click on the arrow at the top right corner of the screen to turn to page 2.
• Read Wilson Metcalf's Health History form that was completed on 1-4-2007.

7. Who do you think filled out the Health History form?

8. Under Section IV, General Health Attitude and Habits, what was Mr. Metcalf's response to the question about how much alcohol he drinks, if any?

9. According to the form, did Mr. Metcalf believe he had a problem with alcohol?

10. On this form, how much coffee does Mr. Metcalf say he drinks?

11. Are Wilson Metcalf's answers on the form consistent with the documentation in his Progress Notes? Explain. If the answers are not consistent, why do you think this may have happened?

12. Why would it have been important for the medical assistant to review this history with Wilson Metcalf?

13. Assume that you interviewed Wilson Metcalf on 1-4-2007 and wrote the Progress Notes on that date. Complete the blank page of the General Health History Questionnaire below by answering the questions correctly for Mr. Metcalf based on the information he provided during the interview.

○   ○

ANDRUS/CLINI-REC ® **HEALTH HISTORY QUESTIONNAIRE**   Chart No. _____

Identification Information   Today's Date _____

Name_____ Date of Birth_____

Occupation _____ Marital Status _____

PART A – PRESENT HEALTH HISTORY

I. CURRENT MEDICAL PROBLEMS

Please list the medical problems for which you came to see the doctor. About when did they begin?

Problems   Date Began

_____   _____
_____   _____
_____   _____

What concerns you most about these problems?

_____
_____

If you are being treated for any other illness or medical problems by another physician, please describe the problems and write the name of the physician or medical facility treating you.

Illness or Medical Problem   Physician or Medical Facility   City

_____   _____   _____
_____   _____   _____

II. MEDICATIONS

Please list all medications you are now taking, including those you buy without a doctor's prescription (such as aspirin, cold tablets or vitamin supplements).

_____   _____   _____
_____   _____   _____

III. ALLERGIES AND SENSITIVITIES

List anything that you are allergic to such as certain foods, medications, dust, chemicals or soaps, household items, pollens, bee stings, etc., and indicate how each affects you.

Allergic To: Effect   Allergic To: Effect

_____   _____   _____   _____
_____   _____   _____   _____

IV. GENERAL HEALTH, ATTITUDE AND HABITS

How is your overall health now?	Health now:	Poor ____	Fair ____	Good ____	Excellent ____
How has it been most of your life?	Health has been:	Poor ____	Fair ____	Good ____	Excellent ____

In the past year:

Has your appetite changed?	Appetite:	Decreased ____	Increased ____	Stayed same ____	
Has your weight changed?	Weight:	Lost ____ lbs.	Gained ____ lbs.	No change ____	
Are you thirsty much of the time?	Thirsty:	No ____	Yes ____		
Has your overall 'pep' changed?	Pep:	Decreased ____	Increased ____	Stayed same ____	

Do you usually have trouble sleeping? Trouble sleeping: No ____ Yes ____

How much do you exercise? Exercise: Little or none ____ Less than I need ____ All I need ____

Do you smoke? Smokes: No ____ Yes ____ If yes, how many years? ____

How many each day? ____ Cigarettes ____ Cigars ____ Pipesfull

Have you ever smoked? Smoked: No ____ Yes ____ If yes, how many years? ____

How many each day? ____ Cigarettes ____ Cigars ____ Pipesfull

Do you drink alcoholic beverages? Alcohol: No ____ Yes ____ I drink ____ Beers ____ Glasses of wine ____ Drinks of hard liquor - per day

Have you ever had a problem with alcohol? Prior problem: No ____ Yes ____

How much coffee or tea do you usually drink? Coffee/Tea: ____ cups of coffee or tea a day

Do you regularly wear seatbelts? Seatbelts: No ____ Yes ____

DO YOU:	Rarely/Never	Occasionally	Frequently	DO YOU:	Rarely/Never	Occasionally	Frequently
Feel nervous?	____	____	____	Ever feel like committing suicide?	____	____	____
Feel depressed?	____	____	____	Feel bored with your life?	____	____	____
Find it hard to make decisions?	____	____	____	Use marijuana?	____	____	____
Lose your temper?	____	____	____	Use 'hard drugs'?	____	____	____
Worry a lot?	____	____	____	Do you want to talk to the doctor about a personal matter? No ____ Yes ____			
Tire easily?	____	____	____				
Have trouble relaxing?	____	____	____				
Have any sexual problems?	____	____	____				

Created and Developed by 'Medical Economics' Professional Systems
Copyright © 1979, 1983 Bibbero Systems International, Inc.   STOCK NO. 19-742-4   8/95   Page 1

C O N F I D E N T I A L

14. Suppose that Mac Wallace (born 10-23-1980) comes to the office stating he has a fever and sore throat. He has had difficulty swallowing and has had pain in his right ear. All of these symptoms have lasted for about 4 days and have become progressively worse each day. He has also run out of blood pressure medicine and wants the prescription to be refilled. Before his throat became sore, his child had a strep throat. Document Mac Wallace's chief complaint on the Progress Notes below.

PATIENT'S NAME		☐ FEMALE ☐ MALE	Date of Birth: / /
DATE	PATIENT VISITS AND FINDINGS		

ALLERGIC TO

ORDER #25-7133-01 • © 1999 BIBBERO SYSTEMS, INC. • PETALUMA, CA   TO REORDER CALL 800-BIBBERO (800-242-2376) OR FAX (800) 242-9330 MFG IN USA   PAGE ____ of ____

15. What subjective symptoms does Mac Wallace report?

16. Which of these subjective symptoms could become objective symptoms following physical examination?

Patient Reception

∽ **Reading Assignment:** Chapter 37—Patient Reception

Patients: Teresa Hernandez, Wilson Metcalf

Objectives:

- Discuss measures to protect the confidentiality of patients in the reception area.
- List information that must be obtained from new patients.
- Describe the proper check-in procedures for new and established patients.
- Discuss procedures necessary to verify whether a patient's insurance will pay for services.
- Describe the steps necessary for replenishing supplies.

Exercise 1

 CD-ROM Activity—Checking Equipment and Supplies

🕐 30 minutes

- Sign in to Mountain View Clinic.
- On the office map, click on **Office Manager** to enter the manager's office. (*Note:* It is not necessary to select a patient to enter this area.)

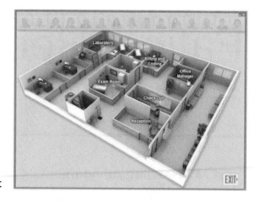

Click on Office Manager.

- Under View, select **Supply Inventory** to review the inventory records.

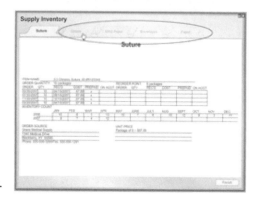

Click on Supply Inventory.

- To view the record for each item in inventory, click on the individual tab headings at the top of the record.

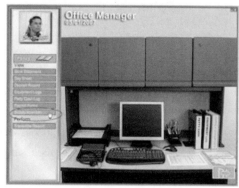

Click on tab headings to view each item.

1. What is the reorder point for sutures?

2. It is currently May 1, 2007, and you need to decide whether or not to order more sutures. As a point of reference, how many packages of sutures were used in May 2006?

3. Should sutures be reordered? If so, how many? If not, why not?

➡ • Click on the tab heading for **EKG Paper** to view that inventory record.

4. When was the last order placed for EKG paper, and how much was ordered?

5. When was this order received?

6. What is the reorder point for EKG paper?

7. How many packs of EKG paper are currently in inventory?

8. Should EKG paper be reordered now? Why or why not? If you reorder, what quantity should be ordered?

➡ • Click **Finish** to return to the Office Manager area.
  • Click the exit arrow and select **Return to Map**.

Exercise 2

CD-ROM Activity—Maintaining Confidentiality

 30 minutes

- Sign in to Mountain View Clinic.
- Select **Teresa Hernandez** from the patient list. (*Note:* If you have exited the program, sign in again to Mountain View Clinic and select Teresa Hernandez from the patient list.)

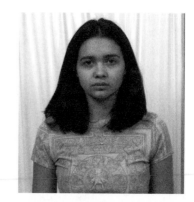

Teresa Hernandez

- On the office map, click on **Reception**.

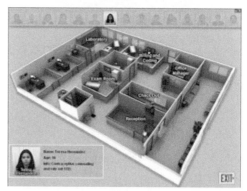

Click on Reception.

- Under the Watch heading, select **Patient Check-In** to view the video.

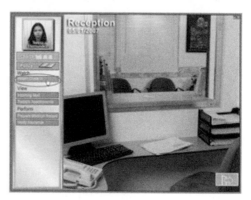

Watch Patient Check-In.

- At the end of the video, click **Close** to return to the Reception desk.

1. As Teresa was checking in, did Kristin take all the necessary steps to protect Teresa's confidential health information? Explain.

2. What additional steps could Kristin have taken to ensure Teresa's privacy was protected?

3. What form was Kristin referring to, and what is the purpose of this form?

4. According to Teresa, she is covered by her father's insurance. Can she request that the insurance company send the EOB for her visit to an address other than the guarantor's? Why or why not?

5. Was the receptionist correct in suggesting that Teresa could provide a different address for mailing insurance statements? Why or why not?

Exercise 3

 CD-ROM Activity—Check-In Procedure for a New Patient

 15 minutes

- For this exercise, you will remain in the Reception area with Teresa as your patient. (*Note:* If you have exited the program, sign in again to Mountain View Clinic, select Teresa Hernandez from the patient list, and go to the Reception area.)
- Under View, select **Today's Appointments** to review the schedule for the day.

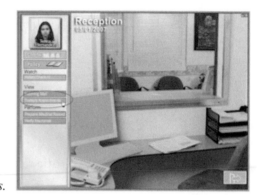

Click on Today's Appointments.

- Locate Teresa Hernandez's name on the schedule.

1. What time is Teresa's scheduled appointment?

2. There is a notation next to Teresa's name in the appointment book. What is the notation, and what does it mean?

 • Click **Finish** to close the Appointment Book and return to the Reception desk.
- Under the **Perform** heading, select **Verify Insurance**.
- Select the appropriate question to ask Teresa.

3. What information does Kristin need to get from Teresa based on her response?

 • Click **Finish** to return to the Reception desk.
- Click the exit arrow and select **Return to Map**.

Exercise 4

 CD-ROM Activity—Check-In Procedure for an Established Patient

 20 minutes

- From the patient list, select **Wilson Metcalf**. (*Note:* If you have exited the program, sign in again to Mountain View Clinic and select Wilson Metcalf from the patient list.)

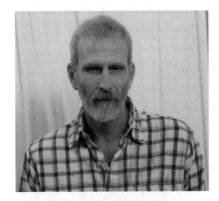

Wilson Metcalf

- On the office map, click on **Reception**.
- Under Watch, select **Patient Check-In** to view the check-in video.
- Stop the video and click **Close** when Kristin closes the window on Mr. Metcalf.

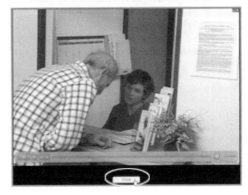

Close the video.

- At the Reception desk, click on **Verify Insurance**.
- Ask the appropriate question of Mr. Metcalf.
- Leave the Verify Insurance window open as you complete the following questions.

1. What information does Kristin need to obtain from Mr. Metcalf based on his response?

2. Using the blank Primary Insurance section of the Patient Information Form below, update Mr. Metcalf's insurance information. (*Note:* The new insurance cards can be viewed in the Verify Insurance window.)

PRIMARY INSURANCE

Person Responsible for Account _____
Last Name   First Name   Initial

Relation to Patient _____ Birthdate _____ Soc. Sec.# _____

Address (if different from patient's) _____ Phone _____

City _____ State _____ Zip _____

Person Responsible Employed by _____ Occupation _____

Business Address _____ Business Phone _____

Insurance Company _____

Contract # _____ Group # _____ Subscriber # _____

Name of other dependents covered under this plan _____

ADDITIONAL INSURANCE

Is patient covered by additional insurance?   ____ Yes ____ No

Subscriber Name _____ Relation to Patient _____ Birthdate _____

Address (if different from patient's) _____ Phone _____

City _____ State _____ Zip _____

Subscriber Employed by _____ Business Phone _____

Insurance Company _____ Soc. Sec.# _____

Contract # _____ Group # _____ Subscriber # _____

Name of other dependents covered under this plan _____

View:

Insurance Card(s)

Patient Information Form

Computer Information

<< Back   Finish

Scheduling Appointments

✐ Reading Assignment: Chapter 40—Scheduling Appointments

Patient: Janet Jones

Objectives:

- Discuss the rationale for providing space in a day's appointment schedule for emergency appointments.
- Explain the need for a matrix on the appointment schedule.
- Describe the role of the Policy Manual in appointment scheduling.
- Explain the importance of verbal communication concerning appointment delays.
- Apply the skills of scheduling appointments in person and by telephone.
- Apply the skills of maintaining the appointment book.
- Identify office policies concerning rescheduling appointments.
- Apply the skills of rescheduling appointments.

Exercise 1

CD-ROM Activity—Using a Specific Daily Appointment Schedule

20 minutes

- Sign in to Mountain View Clinic
- From the patient list, select Janet Jones.

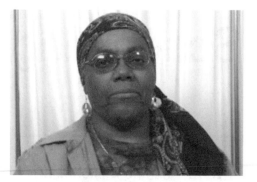

Janet Jones

- On the office map, highlight and click on **Reception**.

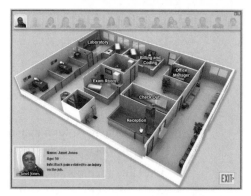

Click on Reception.

- At the Reception desk, click **Today's Appointments** (under the View heading) to open the appointment book. Review the scheduled appointments.

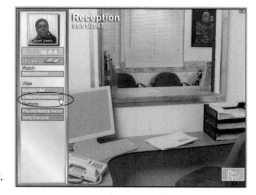

Click on Today's Appointments.

- Click **Finish** to close the appointment book and return to the Reception desk.

1. According to the appointment schedule, what time is Janet Jones' appointment?

2. If Janet Jones signed in at 1:30 p.m., would she have been on time for her appointment? Explain your answer.

- Under the Watch heading, click **Patient Check-In** and watch the video.
- Click **Close** at the end of the video to return to the Reception desk.

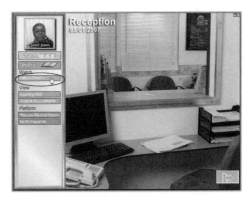

Click on Patient Check-In.

3. Janet Jones is upset when she arrives at the counter. How does Kristin handle the patient in a professional way through verbal and nonverbal communication?

4. Assuming that Ms. Jones checked in at 1:30 p.m., what would have been an appropriate statement for the receptionist to make as the patient checked in to prevent her from becoming so upset?

- At the Reception desk, click on **Policy** to open the office Policy Manual.

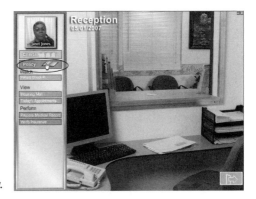

Click on Policy.

• Type "appointment scheduling" in the search bar and click on the magnifying glass.

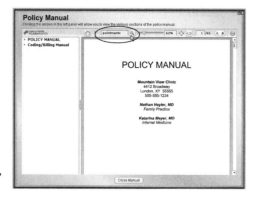

Search for "appointment scheduling."

• Read the section of the Policy Manual on scheduling appointments.

5. What is the length of time needed for an appointment during which a history and physical examination must be completed for a new patient?

6. Why is it necessary to set up a matrix before making appointments?

7. What buffer times are available for emergency appointments?

8. According to the office Policy Manual, what would have been appropriate concerning rescheduling this patient's appointment?

9. Why is it important to identify Workers' Compensation appointments at the time of scheduling rather than at the time of the appointment?

- Click **Close Manual** to return to the Reception desk.
- Leave **Reception** by clicking the exit arrow at the lower right corner of the screen.

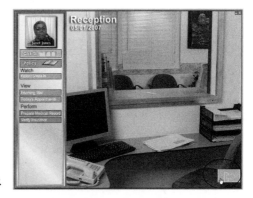

Click the exit arrow.

- At the Summary Menu, select **Return to Map** and continue to the next exercise.

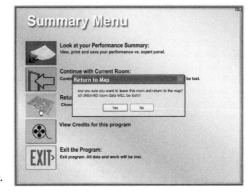

Click on Return to Map.

Exercise 2

 Writing Activity—Adding Appointments to a Schedule

 30 minutes

At the end of the day on April 31, a list of patients needing appointments on May 1 was shown to Dr. Hayler and Dr. Meyer. Both physicians stated that because few patients were currently in the hospital, they would be able to see patients in the clinic earlier than usual the next morning. Dr. Hayler and Dr. Meyer will begin seeing patients at 8:15 a.m. The staff has been informed of the early start.

   1. a. Insert the following appointments for Dr. Hayler onto the morning schedule on the next page.

       (1) Robert Leuker is a patient who has not been to the clinic in 5 years and wants to be seen for a lump in his arm. He has a past history of cancer and needs to be seen ASAP. He should be seen first in the morning so that he can be referred as necessary. He is insured through BlueCross/BlueShield (BC/BS).

       (2) Lindsey Repp needs a follow-up appointment for an earache and recurrent fever. She is insured through Central Health HMO and can be double-booked at the end of the appointment for Louise Parlet.

       (3) John Price, who needs a follow-up appointment for his blood pressure, has Medicare. His blood pressure was low when he took it yesterday, and he feels dizzy. He simply wants Dr. Hayler to reevaluate his medication. He can be seen just before lunch.

5/1/20XX	Dr. Hayler			Dr. Meyer	
Time	Patient Name	Insurance		Patient Name	Insurance
8:00 AM	(Hospital rounds) Joe Smitty - Chem 12, CBC Marsha Brady - Fasting BS			(Hospital Rounds)	
8:15 AM	(Hospital rounds)			(Hospital Rounds) Joanne Crosby, PT, PTT	
8:30 AM	Louise Parlet, Est. Pt New Pregnancy/Pelvic (555) 555-3214	Teachers		Rhea Davison, Est. Pt. Elevated BS, abdominal distention, pelvic (555) 555-5656	None
8:45 AM					
9:00 AM					
9:15 AM					
9:30 AM				Hu Huang, Est. Pt. Severe cough, fever (555) 555-1454	Medicare
9:45 AM	Jade Wong, NP 7 mos well child checkup/ immunization (555) 555-3345	Central Health HMO			
10:00 AM				~~Chris O'Neill - back pain~~ (pt cancelled - resched 5/7) Jesus Santo, Walk-in Leg pain, SOB	None
10:15 AM					
10:30 AM				Jean Deere, Est. Pt. Memory loss, ear pain (555) 555-6361	Medicare
10:45 AM	Tristan Tsosie, Est. Pt. Suture Removal (555) 555-1515	Blue Cross/ Blue Shield			
11:00 AM					
11:15 AM				Wilson Metcalf, Est. Pt. N/V, abdominal pain, difficulty urinating - (555) 555-3311	Medicare
11:30 AM	LUNCH				
11:45 AM					
12:00 PM					
12:15 PM	Renee Anderson, NP Annual GYN Exam (555) 555-3331	Blue Cross/ Blue Shield			

b. After completing Dr. Hayler's appointments, add the following appointments for Dr. Meyer in the morning, using the same schedule on the previous page.

(1) Catherine Lake needs a follow-up appointment for pyelonephritis. She forgot to make her follow-up appointment when she was last seen. Ms. Lake is going out of town for 2 weeks and needs to see Dr. Meyer before leaving. Her insurance coverage is through BC/BS. Dr. Meyer will see her at the earliest appointment time.

(2) Lucille Meryl needs to be seen for a follow-up to a thyroid test. Dr. Meyer wants to see her as a double-booking at the end of the appointment for Rhea Davison. Her insurance is through Drake.

(3) An established patient, Simon Reed, calls at 11:30 a.m. to tell you that he has some chest pain, and even though he has an appointment for tomorrow, he does not think he should wait. When you discuss this with Dr. Meyer, she tells you to book him ASAP. Mr. Reed, who has BC/BS insurance, tells you that it will take him about 20 minutes to get to the office.

2. You must now call John Price to inform him that Dr. Hayler will see him just before lunch. Write the information below that Mr. Price will need to be told. Why did Dr. Hayler need to be contacted before making the appointment for Mr. Price?

3. You must also call Lucille Meryl to inform her that Dr. Meyer wants to see her about her test results. What information do you need to provide, and how would you answer her when she questions why she needs to be seen so quickly?

Exercise 3

CD-ROM Activity—Preparing an Appointment Schedule

30 minutes

- In this exercise we will continue with Janet Jones' visit. (*Note:* If you have exited the program, sign in again to Mountain View Clinic and select Janet Jones from the patient list.
- On the office map, click on **Check Out**.

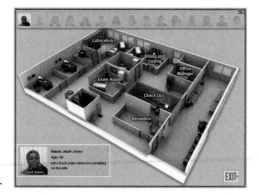

Click on Check Out.

- At the Check Out desk, click **Encounter Form** under the View heading.

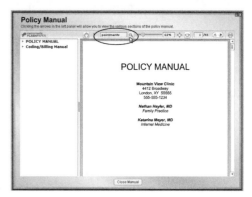

Click on Encounter Form.

1. What is the date that Janet Jones should return to the clinic for a follow-up appointment?

2. How much time should be allotted to the follow-up appointment for Ms. Jones?

Complete the following activities using the appointment sheets on the next two pages.

(1) Set up the appointment sheet for the date that Janet Jones is to return for her follow-up visit.

(2) Using the information in the Policy Manual, set up the matrix for that day. (*Note:* If you need to review this, return to the Policy Manual, type "hours of operation" in the search bar, and click on the magnifying glass.)

(3) Before entering an appointment for Janet Jones, add an appointment at 11:00 a.m. for Kay Soto (an established patient) with Dr. Meyer. Ms. Soto has been prescribed a weight loss program and is coming in for a weight check. Her insurance is through Metro HMO.

Continue adding appointments to the schedule using the list provided at the top of page 318.

3.

Appointment Book, Page 1

_/_/20XX	Dr. Hayler		Dr. Meyer	
Time	Patient Name	Insurance	Patient Name	Insurance
8:00 AM				
8:15 AM				
8:30 AM				
8:45 AM				
9:00 AM				
9:15 AM				
9:30 AM				
9:45 AM				
10:00 AM				
10:15 AM				
10:30 AM				
10:45 AM				
11:00 AM				
11:15 AM				
11:30 AM				
11:45 AM				
12:00 PM				
12:15 PM				

4.

Appointment Book, Page 2

/ /20XX	Dr. Hayler		Dr. Meyer	
Time	Patient Name	Insurance	Patient Name	Insurance
12:30 PM				
12:45 PM				
1:00 PM				
1:15 PM				
1:30 PM				
1:45 PM				
2:00 PM				
2:15 PM				
2:30 PM				
2:45 PM				
3:00 PM				
3:15 PM				
3:30 PM				
3:45 PM				
4:00 PM				
4:15 PM				
4:30 PM				
4:45 PM				
5:00 PM				

Continue your scheduling by adding the following appointments or adjustments to the forms on the previous two pages.

(4) George Smith, age 15, is to be seen by Dr. Hayler for a football injury the night before. He has State Agricultural Insurance and is an existing patient. George needs to be seen as early as possible so that he can go to school.

(5) Callie Agree, a new patient, is to be seen for a possible sinus infection. She has Medicare and will be accompanied by her daughter. The daughter prefers to see Dr. Meyer in the midmorning so that her mother will have time to dress.

(6) Sophie Coats, age 6 months, is an established patient who will be seen by Dr. Hayler for a well-baby visit. She is due to have immunizations at this visit. Her mother prefers to have an appointment as early in the morning as possible. Sophie is covered by her father's insurance with Banker's Health.

(7) Mamie Mack, age 18, is an established patient who needs a physical for college. She prefers to be seen by Dr. Hayler. Either late morning or early afternoon is better for her since she is still in school. She is covered through George Allen Insurance at her mother's place of employment.

(8) Kay Soto calls to cancel her appointment for the day because she has to leave town to take care of her ill mother. She does not want to reschedule at this time.

(9) Make the appointment for Janet Jones for her follow-up visit.

(10) Dr. Hayler will need to leave at 11:15 for a dental appointment but will be back in the afternoon. Mark this on the appointment sheet.

(11) Dr. Meyer is scheduled to be off the afternoon of this day. Mark this on the appointment sheet.

5. What are the necessary procedures for canceling Kay Soto's appointment?
   a. Erase the canceled appointment and tell Ms. Soto that there will be a charge because she did not give 24 hours' notice.
   b. Cross out the appointment (using the office-preferred writing implement) and record the cancellation in the patient medical record.
   c. Report the cancellation to Dr. Meyer.
   d. Tell Kay Soto that she must reschedule this appointment today for continued medical care.

LESSON 30

Filing Medical Records

/OᴿᏫ **Reading Assignment:** Chapter 41—Medical Records Management

Patients: All

Objectives:

- Alphabetize patient names for efficiency in filing medical records.
- List the necessary steps needed to prepare a medical record for filing.
- Describe the use of outguides, colored file folders, color-coded name labels, and aging labels.
- Incorporate correct labeling to provide ease of filing.
- Describe the differences in alphabetic and numeric filing.
- Discuss the need to purge older medical records.
- Discuss means for finding displaced medical records.
- Discuss the importance of using correct filing techniques for time management.

319

Exercise 1

 CD-ROM Activity—Preparing Patient Medical Records for Filing

 50 minutes

- Sign in to Mountain View Clinic.
- One at a time, select each patient from the patient list (moving from left to right) and record his or her name in the table in question 1 below.

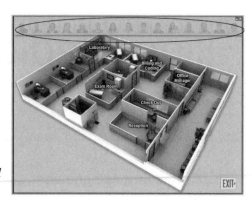

Select each patient and record his or her name in the table below.

1. Record the names of the Mountain View Clinic patients in the first and third columns of the table below. (*Note:* Fill in all of column 1 first; then continue at the top of column 3.)

Patient Name/ NP or Est. Pt.	First Date of Service; Last Date of Service	Patient Name/ NP or Est. Pt.	First Date of Service; Last Date of Service

• Now click again on any patient in the patient list. Then on the office map, click on **Reception**. At the Reception desk, click on **Today's Appointments** to view the day's schedule. Find each patient's name and then indicate next to that patient's name on the table in question 1 whether he or she is a new patient (NP) or an established patient (Est. Pt.) (*Note:* You will return to fill in the remaining columns of the table later in this exercise.)

Click on Today's Appointments.

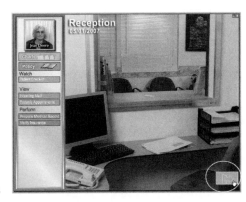

2. With the Today's Appointments window still open, make a list below of the patients Dr. Hayler is to see in the morning. List these patients in the correct order for their appointments and note whether the medical record can be pulled from the files of established patients or whether a new record should be prepared.

3. What medical records will need to be pulled from the files for Dr. Meyer's morning patients? Will any of these patients need to have a new record prepared? List these patients and their record needs below (in the order of their appointment times).

 • Click **Finish** to close the appointment book and return to the Reception desk.

• Click the exit arrow in right lower corner of screen.

Click the exit arrow.

- From the Summary Menu, click on **Return to Map**; then click **Yes** to return to the office map and select another patient.

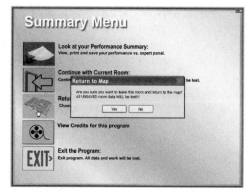

Click on Return to Map.
When prompted, click Yes.

- Beginning with the first patient on the left in the patient list, open each patient's chart, click on the **Patient Medical Information** tab, and select **Progress Notes**. Based on what you find, record each patient's first and last dates of service in columns 2 and 4 in the table in question 1. (*Note:* New patients will not have any forms in their chart. Use today's virtual date, 5-1-07, as their first date of service; there will be no "last date of service" for new patients.)

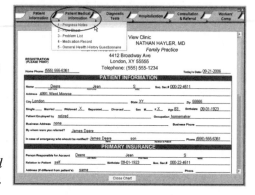

Click on Progress Notes and find
the first and last dates of service.

- When you have recorded the date(s) for the first patient, click **Close Chart**; then click the exit arrow.
- From the Summary Menu, click on **Return to Map**.
- Select your next patient, open the chart, and record the date(s) in the table.
- Continue these steps for each patient until you have completed the table in question 1.

4. Using the table in question 1 as a reference, list the patients' names in alphabetic order in the left column below. In the right column indicate whether the medical records for each patient will be available in the file cabinet of established patients or whether the record will have to be organized and placed in the correct position as a new medical record.

Alphabetic List of Patients   **New or Established Record?**

5. As you pull the medical records for established patients, you will need to change the year on their medical records (unless the patient has already been seen in the current year). List the established patients below and indicate what year will need to be relabeled on their medical record (if this applies).

Name of Established Patient   **Year That Will Need to Be Relabled**

6. At the end of the morning, the medical records need to be filed correctly to prevent loss and to ensure proper time management. Below, list in alphabetic order the names of patients who had morning appointments today and whose records will need to be refiled.

7. Which of the following would *not* be used to help prevent misfiling of medical records?
   a. Colored letter tabs for use with names
   b. Colored tabs for the last year seen in office
   c. Outguides
   d. Alphabet tabs in the filing system

8. The two filing systems most often used in a medical office are _____ and

   _____ filing.

Written Communications

✎ **Reading Assignment:** Chapter 42—Written Communications
Chapter 43—Mail

Patient: Wilson Metcalf

Objectives:

- Prepare letters in response to the mail received.
- Use correct grammar, spelling, and formatting techniques in letter writing.
- Use correct medical terminology as appropriate.
- Answer mail appropriately and promptly.
- Transcribe medical records.

Exercise 1

CD-ROM Activity—Composing a Letter for an NSF Check

🕐 30 minutes

- Sign in to Mountain View Clinic.
- From the patient list, select **Wilson Metcalf**.

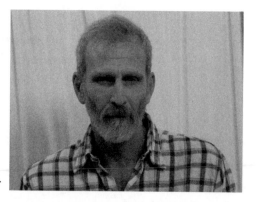

Wilson Metcalf

- On the office map, highlight and click on **Reception** to enter the Reception area.

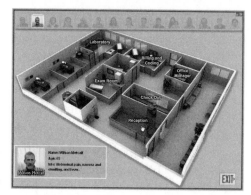

Click on Reception.

- Under the View heading, select **Incoming Mail** to view the mail received by the clinic.

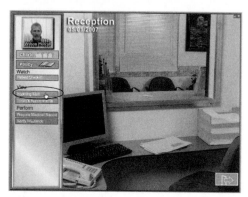

Click on Incoming Mail.

- From the list of mail at the top of the screen, click on **7** to view that piece of mail.

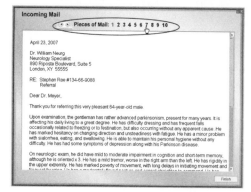

Click on 7.

→ • Your next task will be to compose a letter to the patient regarding the NSF check. Leave the Incoming Mail window open to use for a reference.

1. Below, write your letter to the patient about the NSF check, using an acceptable format. Be sure your message conveys the need to handle this matter within a certain number of days. Include the service charge and make it clear that no further checks will be accepted for this patient's medical care at Mountain View Clinic. This should be prepared for a signature by the office manager.

Mountain View Clinic

4412 Broadway / London, XY 55555 / Phone: (555) 555-1234 / Fax (555) 555-1239

Nathan Hayler, MD - Family Practice / Katarina Meyer, MD - Internal Medicine

Exercise 2

  CD-ROM Activity—Composing a Letter in Response to an Inaccurate Accounts Payable

15 minutes

- We will continue working with the Incoming Mail window. (*Note:* If you have exited the program, sign in again to Mountain View Clinic and select Wilson Metcalf as your patient. Then go to Reception and select Incoming Mail under View.)
- From the list of mail at the top of the screen, click on **10** to read the letter from Summer Oxygen Company.
- Click **Finish** to return to the Reception Desk.

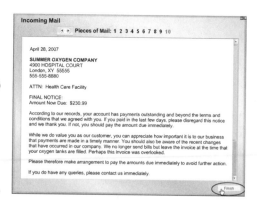

Click on Finish.

- Click the exit arrow to leave the Reception area.
- On the Summary Menu, click **Return to Map**.

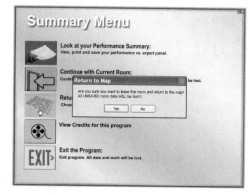

Click Return to Map.

- On the office map, highlight and click on **Office Manager** to enter the manager's office.

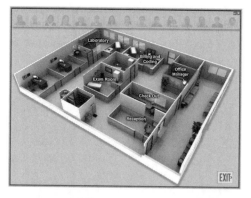

Click on Office Manager.

- Under the View heading, click on **Bank Statement** to view the Clinic's most recent statement from the bank.

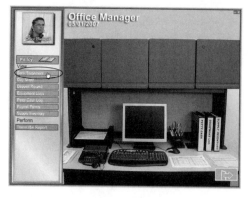

Click on Bank Statement.

→ • Select the **Check Ledger** tab to review the most recent checks written by Mountain View Clinic.

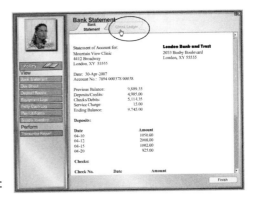

Click on Check Ledger.

1. There was a payment made to Summer Oxygen Company for $230.99.

   a. According to the check ledger, what was the date the payment was made?

   b. What was the check number?

→ • Click on the **Bank Statement** tab to review the account activity for April 2007.

   2. Did check #1230 for $230.99 clear the account, according to the bank statement?

→ • Compose a rough draft for a letter to the oxygen supply company in response to the claim that the invoice has not been paid. Be sure to include in the correspondence that a copy of the canceled check is enclosed with the letter.

• Click **Finish** to return to the manager's office.

3. Below, write your letter to the oxygen company using an acceptable format. Be sure your message includes all information needed to clear the accounts payable. This should be prepared for signature by the office manager.

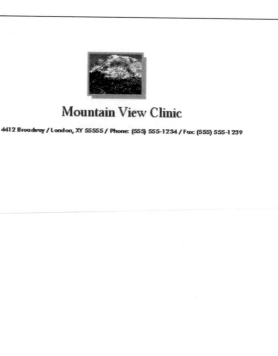

Mountain View Clinic

4412 Broadway / London, XY 55555 / Phone: (555) 555-1234 / Fax (555) 555-1239

Nathan Hayler, MD - Family Practice / Katarina Meyer, MD - Internal Medicine

Exercise 3

 CD-ROM Activity—Medical Transcription

 30 minutes

- Still in the Office Manager's area, click on **Transcribe Report** to access the dictated report.

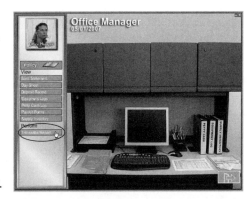

Click on Transcribe Report.

- Review the instructions on how to operate the player and transcribe the discharge report as dictated, using the dates on the recording.
- Be sure that you use the correct format, grammar, style, and medical terminology.
- Click **Print** for a hard copy of your transcription. Click **Finish** to close the player.

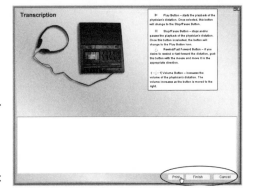

Click Finish to close the player.

Managing Practice Finances

Reading Assignment: Chapter 44—Managing Practice Finances
Chapter 47—Billing and Collections

Patients: All

Objectives:

- Post daily entries on the day sheet and prepare bank deposits at the end of the day.
- Process credit balances, NSF checks, and checks from collection agencies.
- Perform billing and collections procedures.
- Process credit balances and complete necessary steps to process a refund, including preparation of a check.
- Reconcile a bank statement.
- Maintain a petty cash fund.
- Discuss the maintenance of records for accounting and banking purposes.
- Discuss the importance of managing accounts payable promptly.

Exercise 1

  CD-ROM Activity—Posting Charges to Ledger Cards

30 minutes

- Sign in to Mountain View Clinic.
- Select **Jade Wong** from the patient list.

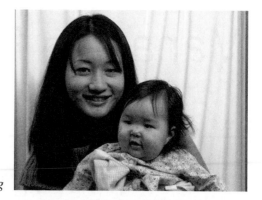

Jade Wong

- On the office map, highlight and click on **Billing and Coding**.

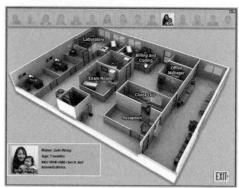

Click on Billing and Coding.

- In the Billing and Coding office, select **Encounter Form** to review the services that will be billed for Jade's visit.

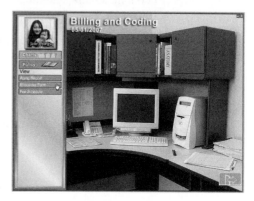

Select Encounter Form.

1. a. Using the Encounter Form for Jade Wong, begin completing the blank ledger card below.
   b. In the column marked Professional Service, list each individual service provided, but do not enter any fee or balance information.
   c. After the last service has been entered, be sure to record that the co-pay was collected and enter the amount in the Payment column.

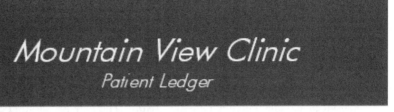

Patient Name:
Insurance Type:

Date	Professional Service	Fee ($)	Payment ($)	Adj. ($)	Prev. Bal. ($)	New Balance ($)
Totals						

→ • Click **Finish** to return to Billing and Coding.
  • Now click on **Fee Schedule** to review the amount Mountain View Clinic charges for various services and procedures.

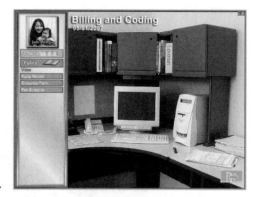

Click on Fee Schedule.

• Again using the ledger card on the previous page, fill in the fees charged for the listed services and calculate the balances. (*Note:* The balance should be adjusted line by line as each service or payment is added or subtracted.)

2. After filling in the services, charges, and payments for Jade's current visit, should the ledger card be totaled as indicated at the bottom of the card? Explain your answer.

→ • Click **Finish** to close the Fee Schedule; then click the exit arrow to leave Billing and Coding.

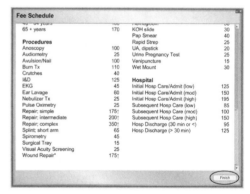

Click Finish.

• On the Summary Menu, click on **Return to Map** and continue to the next exercise.

Exercise 2

 CD-ROM Activity—Posting Entries to a Day Sheet

 60 minutes

1. In this activity you will post charges and payments for the patients who were seen in the office today.

   a. In the Patient Name column on the blank day sheet on the next page, list the patients in the following order: Jade Wong, Louise Parlet, Hu Huang, Rhea Davison, Jesus Santo, Jean Deere, Tristan Tsosie, Wilson Metcalf, Renee Anderson, Jose Imero, Shaunti Begay, Janet Jones, Kevin McKinzie, John R. Simmons, and Teresa Hernandez.

   b. Select Jade Wong from the patient list. Then click on **Check Out** on the office map. Once in the Check Out area, open the **Encounter Form**.

   c. Using one line per patient, complete each column on the day sheet using the Total Charges, Previous Balance, and Amount Received information listed on the Encounter Form. Refer back to the ledger card in Exercise 1 to confirm your totals. (*Note:* Unlike the ledger card, the Professional Service column on the day sheet is a summary description of the visit.)

   d. For the purposes of this exercise, also make a note next to each patient's name to indicate whether the patient paid by cash, check, or credit card. If payment was made by check, include the check number.

   e. Repeat the above steps by selecting each patient and opening his or her Encounter Form at Check Out. As you finish each patient's portion of the day sheet, click **Finish** to close the Encounter Form. Click the exit arrow to leave Check Out and choose **Return to Map** to select the next patient.

   f. When you finish recording the information for the last patient on the list, remain at the office map to continue with this exercise.

Mountain View Clinic
Daysheet

Date	Professional Service	Fee	Payment	Adjustment	New Balance	Old Balance	Patient's Name	Distribution Dr. Hayler	Distribution Dr. Meyer
TOTALS								TOTALS	

- From the office map, click on **Reception**.
  (*Note:* Your selected patient should be Teresa
  Hernandez, the last patient on the list in
  question 1.)
- At the Reception desk, click on **Incoming Mail**
  to view the day's correspondence.

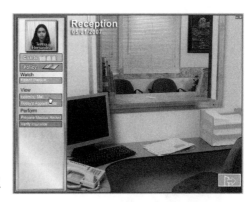

Click Incoming Mail.

2. a. View each piece of incoming mail; then on the blank day sheet on the next page, record
      any payments *received* by the clinic and any charges *paid* by the clinic in the appropriate
      columns.
   b. Be sure to include a description of the payment/charge and the patient's name.
   c. For the purposes of this exercise, make a note of the bank and check number next to the
      name of any patient who paid by check.
   d. To complete the remaining columns, first click **Finish** to close the mail.
   e. Next, click the exit arrow and **Return to Map**.
   f. Click on **Office Manager** and then on **Day Sheet** (under View) to find any previous bal-
      ance information. Then recalculate the balance and record in the New Balance column.

Mountain View Clinic
Daysheet

Date	Professional Service	Fee	Payment	Adjustment	New Balance	Old Balance	Patient's Name	Distribution Dr. Hayler	Distribution Dr. Meyer
TOTALS								TOTALS	

• Click **Finish** and continue to the next exercise.

Exercise 3

 Writing Activity—Preparing a Bank Deposit

15 minutes

1. Using the information you recorded in the day sheet in Exercise 2, you will now prepare a bank deposit (both front and back) for the accounts receivable for the day. Be sure the total on the deposit slip balances with the total of receivables on the day sheet.

   Below, complete the front side of the deposit slip.

DEPOSIT SLIP

Clarion National Bank
90 Grape Vine Road
London, XY 55555-0001

Mountain View Clinic
4412 Broadway
London, XY 55555

Date: _____

_____
SIGN HERE IN TELLER'S PRESENCE FOR CASH RECEIVED

CASH			TOTAL
	Currency	$	
	Coin	$	
	Total Cash		$
CHECKS	See other side for detail		$
- CASH REC'D			$
NET DEPOSIT			$

---

2. Below, complete the back portion of the bank deposit slip. (*Note:* The bank number cannot be obtained from the day sheet. For the purposes of this exercise, use the check number as a substitute.)

BANK DEPOSIT DETAIL

PAYMENTS

BANK NUMBER	BY CHECK OR PMO		BY COIN OR CURRENCY		CREDIT CARD	
TOTALS						
CURRENCY						
COIN						
CHECKS						
CREDIT CARDS						
TOTAL RECEIPTS						
LESS CREDIT CARD $						
TOTAL DEPOSIT						
DEPOSIT DATE_____						

Exercise 4

 CD-ROM Activity—Processing Credit Balances

 20 minutes

- Remain in the manager's office and click on **Day Sheet**. (*Note:* If you have exited the manager's office and are at the office map, click on **Office Manager** and then click on **Day Sheet**.)

    1. Two patients listed on the day sheet have overpaid, resulting in a credit balance. What are the names of these two patients, and how much money should be refunded to each of them?

    2. The day sheet indicates that _____ has already been sent a

       refund, but the refund for _____ still needs to be processed.

    3. Using the blank check below, process the outstanding refund for payment.

173975		
DATE: _____		
TO: _____		
FOR: _____		
BALANCE BROUGHT FORWARD		
DEPOSITS		
BALANCE		
AMT THIS CHECK		
BALANCE CARRIED FORWARD		

MOUNTAIN VIEW CLINIC   173975
4412 Broadway
London, XY 55555   94-72/1224
                                   Date: _____

Pay to the order of: _____

_____ *Dollars*

Clarion National Bank
        Member FDIC
90 Grape Vine Road   _____
London, XY 55555-0001   *Authorized Signature*

||■ 005503 ||■ ⁴⁴6782011 ||■ 678800470

➡ - Click **Finish** to return to the manager's office.

Exercise 5

 CD-ROM Activity—Maintaining Petty Cash Fund

 30 minutes

• In the manager's office, click on **Petty Cash**. (*Note:* If you have exited the manager's office and are at the office map, click on **Office Manager** and select **Petty Cash**.)

1. Petty cash was used to pay for the mailing of a certified letter. What is the receipt number and date from this transaction?

2. On 5-1-07, the administrative medical assistant was asked to obtain soft drinks for an office celebration to be held that afternoon. She bought these at Sav-A-Grocery for the amount of $24.56. She also mailed a large package at the post office. The cost for mailing the package was $15.08. Using the form below, fill out the first petty cash voucher.

```
Date: _____                      No.: _109_
Amount: [        ]
                      PETTY CASH VOUCHER

For: _____


Charge to: _____
_____

Approved by: _____        Received by: _____


_____        _____
Authorized Signature
```

3. Now fill out the second petty cash voucher.

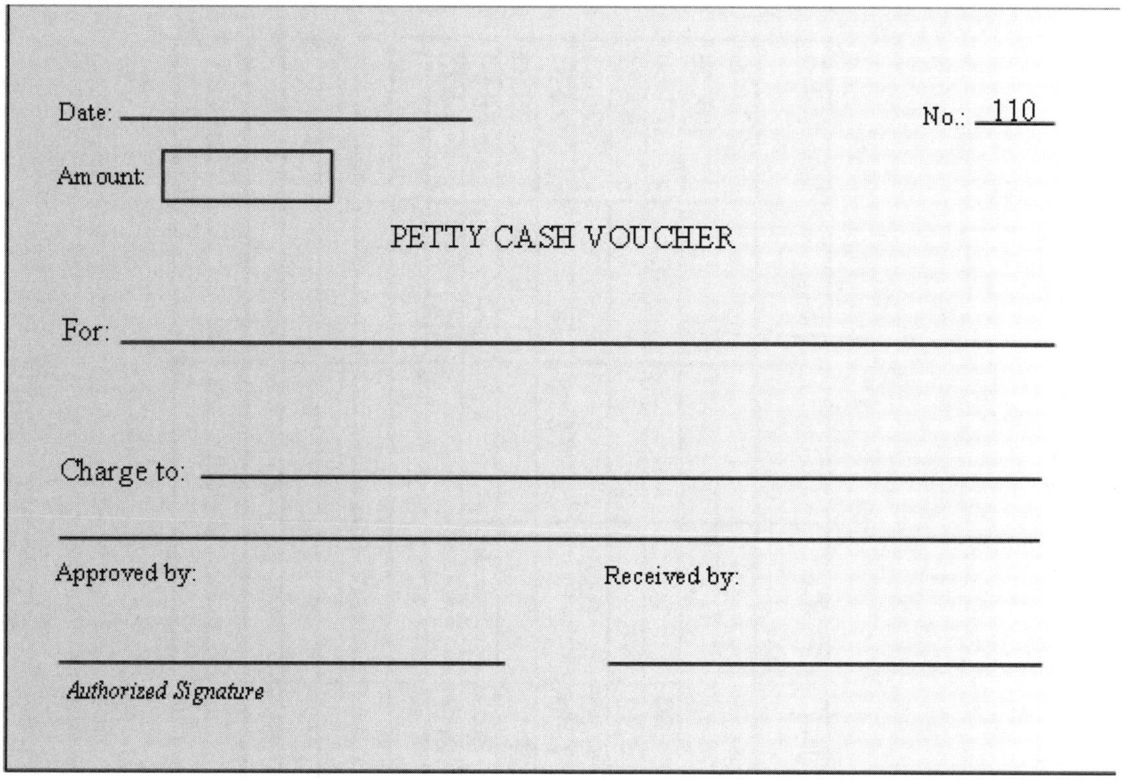

Date: _____   No.: __110__

Amount: [   ]

PETTY CASH VOUCHER

For: _____

Charge to: _____

_____

Approved by: Received by:

_____   _____

Authorized Signature

4. Using the completed petty cash vouchers from questions 2 and 3, update the petty cash log below. Be sure to distribute the expenses to the proper expense column.

NO.	DATE	DESCRIPTION	AMOUNT	OFFICE EXP.	AUTO.	MISC.	BALANCE
	2/16/2007	Fund Established (check #217)					200.00
101	2/24/2007	Certified Letter	3.74	3.74			196.26
102	3/1/2007	Staff Meeting/Lunch	24.60			24.60	171.66
103	3/6/2007	Coffee	4.32			4.32	167.34
104	3/8/2007	Tympanic Thermometer	38.00	38.00			129.34
105	3/8/2007	Parking Fee	6.00		6.00		123.34
106	4/1/2007	Staff Meeting/Lunch	27.43			27.43	95.91
107	4/13/2007	Miscellaneous Supplies	9.01	9.01			86.90
108	4/21/2007	Patient Birthday Cards	12.17	12.17			74.73

5. Office policy states that petty cash should be replenished when the amount falls below $50. Use the blank check below to replenish the petty cash fund to the full $200 balance as required by the office policy. Then, using the updated petty cash log in question 4, verify the petty cash fund balances by totaling all the columns and add this transaction to the log.

173976

DATE: _____

TO: _____

FOR: _____

ACCOUNT NO. _____

AMOUNT PAID $ _____

MOUNTAIN VIEW CLINIC
4412 Broadway
London, XY 55555

173976

94-72/1224

Date: _____

Pay to the order of: _____

_____ Dollars

Clarion National Bank
Member FDIC
90 Grape Vine Road
London, XY 55555-0001

_____
Authorized Signature

⑆005503⑆ ⑈4678201⑆ 678800470

→ • Click **Finish** to return to the manager's office.
 • Click the exit arrow; from the Summary Menu, select **Return to Map**.
 • On the office map, select **Jose Imero** from the patient list and click on **Check Out**.
 • At the Check Out desk, select **Patient Check Out** (under Watch) to view the video.

6. What are the ethical implications of Kristin asking another medical assistant for money from petty cash?

→ • Click **Close** to return to the Check Out desk.
 • Click the exit arrow; from the Summary Menu, select **Return to Map**.

Exercise 6

  CD-ROM Activity—Managing Accounts Payable

30 minutes

- Using any patient from the patient list, click on **Reception** on the office map. (*Note:* You may continue with Jose Imero from the previous exercise.)
- Select **Incoming Mail** (under View) and review pieces 8 and 9.

1. True or False:

   a. _____ When accounts payable arrive, the date for payment with discounts should be noted.

   b. _____ It really does not matter what day of the month an accounts payable payment is made, as long as it is paid before the next billing cycle.

   c. _____ Invoices should be marked with the date and check number, as well as the initials of the person preparing the check.

   d. _____ All accounts payables should be checked against invoices and packing slips before payment is made.

   e. _____ All vendors will present invoices before payment is due.

2. Which of the following information does the accounts payable person need to have to correctly process and post the payment of the invoices (pieces 8 and 9 of the incoming mail)? Select all that apply.

   _____ Invoice number

   _____ Company name

   _____ Name of customer service representative

   _____ Date of check

   _____ Account number

   _____ Company address

   _____ Company phone number

   _____ Name of the company's bank

   _____ Company's bank account number

   _____ Type of expense

   _____ Amount of the check

   _____ Invoice date

   _____ Check number

- Click **Finish** to close the mail and return to the Reception desk.
- Click the exit arrow; from the Summary Menu, select **Return to Map**.

Exercise 7

 CD-ROM Activity—Reconciling a Bank Statement

 30 minutes

In today's mail, the clinic's bank statement arrives. This is found in the manager's office. She is extremely busy and asks that you take the time to reconcile the statement for her.

- On the office map, click on **Office Manager** to enter the manager's office. (*Note:* It is not necessary to select a patient to enter this area.)
- From the menu on the left, select **Bank Statement**.

1. a. Using the check ledger below, review the bank statement and check off each deposit, check, withdrawal, ATM transaction, or credit listed on the statement.
   b. If the statement shows any interest paid to the account, any service charges, bank fees, automatic payments, or ATM transactions withdrawn from the account that are not listed on the check ledger, make an entry for those items now and recalculate the account balance in the ledger.

No.	Date	Description	Payment/ Debit	Ref	Deposit/ Credit	Balance
1216	3/5/2007	Rocke Medical	$625.00			$9,264.35
1217	3/5/2007	Wal Store	$38.46			$9,225.89
1218	3/6/2007	Lorenz Equipment	$1,006.00			$8,219.89
1219	3/8/2007	Office Station	$199.43			$8,020.46
	3/10/2007	Dep. Daily Trans			$1,050.00	$10,833.46
1220	3/10/2007	West Electric	$93.99			$7,926.47
	3/12/2007	Dep. Daily Trans			$2,008.00	$9,934.47
1221	3/12/2007	Office Depot	$102.01			$9,832.46
1222	3/12/2007	Video Inc.	$49.00			$9,783.46
	3/15/2007	Dep. Daily Trans			$1,002.00	$11,835.46
1223	3/17/2007	Bonus	$200.00			$12,560.46
1224	3/17/2007	Bonus	$200.00			$12,360.46
1225	3/17/2007	Bonus	$200.00			$12,160.46
	3/20/2007	Dep. Daily Trans			$925.00	$12,760.46
1226	3/21/2007	Jamison Medical	$2,024.20			$10,136.26
1227	3/22/2007	Healthy Living Magazine	$32.95			$10,103.31
1228	3/22/2007	Greater London Electric	$422.00			$9,681.31
1229	3/24/2007	Office Station	$344.70			$9,336.61
1230	3/25/2007	Summer Oxygen	$230.99			$9,105.62
	3/27/2007	Dep. Daily Trans			$1,550.00	$10,655.62

2. Now complete the bank reconciliation worksheet below.

THIS WORKSHEET IS PROVIDED TO HELP YOU BALANCE YOUR ACCOUNT

1. Go through your register and mark each check, withdrawal, Express ATM transaction, payment, deposit or other credit listed on your statement. Be sure that your register shows any interest paid into your account, and any service charges, bank fees, automatic payments, or Express Transfers withdrawn from your account during this statement period.

2. Using the chart below, list any outstanding checks, Express ATM withdrawals, payments or any other withdrawals (including any from previous months) that are listed in your register but are not shown on this statement.

3. Balance your account by filling in the spaces below.

ITEMS OUTSTANDING	
NUMBER	**AMOUNT**
TOTAL	

ENTER

The NEW BALANCE shown on this statement ------------------------------ $ _____ __

ADD

Any deposits listed in your register or $ _____ __
transfers into your account which are $ _____ __
not shown on this statement $ _____ __
                         +$ _____ __

             TOTAL------------------------------------+ $ _____ __

CALCULATE THE SUBTOTAL --- $ _____ __

SUBTRACT

The total outstanding checks and
Withdrawals from the chart at the left --- $ _____ __

CALCULATE THE ENDING BALANCE

This amount should be the same as
The current balance shown in your
Check register --- $ _____ __

Exercise 8

 Writing Activity—Maintaining Financial Records

15 minutes

1. True or False:

   a. _____ All financial records may be discarded after 7 years.

   b. _____ If financial records are discarded early, legal implications are possible.

   c. _____ All financial records should be kept in an active file for 7 years.

   d. _____ The office Policy Manual should provide the guidelines for record retention.

   e. _____ When financial records are stored, the storage boxes should be labeled and stored in logical order.

   f. _____ The medical assistant should obtain the physician's permission before destroying any records.

   g. _____ All financial records must be maintained for the same time limit.

Procedural Coding (E&M and HCPCS)

⌒∞ **Reading Assignment:** Chapter 45—Medical Coding
- Procedural Evaluation and Management and HCPCS Coding

Patients: Jean Deere, Wilson Metcalf, Teresa Hernandez

Objectives:

- Describe the type of codes included in each section of the Current Procedural Terminology (CPT) Manual.
- Assign correct CPT codes to services and/or procedures provided to selected patients.
- Identify when HCPCS level II codes should be used.
- Demonstrate how to locate an accurate HCPCS level II code.

Exercise 1

 CD-ROM Activity—CPT Coding Assignment 1

 15 minutes

- Sign in to Mountain View Clinic.
- Select **Jean Deere** from the patient list.

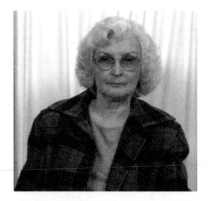

Jean Deere

- Click on **Billing and Coding** on the office map

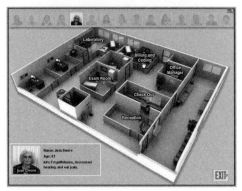

Click on Billing and Coding.

- Once you are in the Billing and Coding office, click on **Encounter Form**.

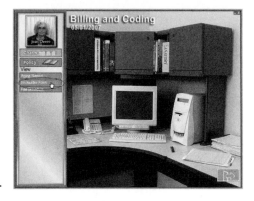

Click on Encounter Form.

1. Ms. Deere is an established patient, and her office visit is a Level IV visit. What is the correct E&M code for this visit level?

2. The procedures/services provided to Ms. Deere today include (1) ear lavage; (2) UA, dipstick; and (3) pulse oximetry. Using the most recent CPT-4 coding manual, provide the correct codes for these three services/procedures.

3. _____ True or False: The procedures/services listed on the Encounter Form for Ms. Deere on this date correspond with those documented in the medical chart notes.

4. Suppose Dr. Meyers admits Ms. Deere to the hospital. What is the E&M code for Dr. Meyer's admission and initial hospital care for moderate complexity?

5. What code would be used for Dr. Meyers' subsequent hospital visits (moderate complexity) to Ms. Deere?
   a. 99222
   b. 99232
   c. 99233
   d. 99238

6. Assume that while Ms. Deere is in the hospital, tests indicate a heart problem, so Dr. Meyers calls in cardiologist, Dr. Hudson. Dr. Hudson's inpatient consultation includes a comprehensive history, a comprehensive evaluation, and medical decision making of moderate complexity. What is the correct E&M code for Dr. Hudson's consultation?

7. Dr. Meyers spends 20 minutes with Ms. Deere on the last day of her hospitalization, which

   includes her discharge. The correct code would be _____.

→ • Close Ms. Deere's chart, click the exit arrow, and select **Return to Map**.

Exercise 2

  CD-ROM Activity—CPT Coding Assignment 2

🕐 15 minutes

- From the patient list, choose **Wilson Metcalf**. (*Note:* If you have exited the program, sign in again to Mountain View Clinic and select Wilson Metcalf from the patient list.)

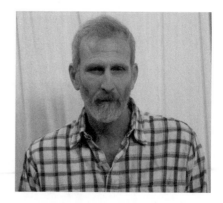

Wilson Metcalf

- Click on **Billing and Coding** on the office map.

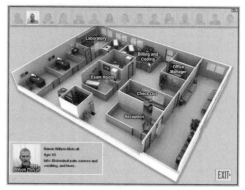

Click on Billing and Coding.

- In the Billing and Coding office, click on **Charts**.
- Click on the **Patient Medical Information** tab and choose **1-Progress Notes**.
- Review the Progress Notes before answering the next questions.

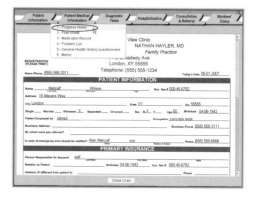

Click on 1-Progress Notes.

1. Were any laboratory tests completed for Mr. Metcalf on 05/01/2007? If so, list and code each test.

2. Besides the exam, were any procedures performed on 05-01-2007? If so, list and code each.

3. We know that Mr. Metcalf was subsequently admitted to the hospital. Let's look at a hypothetical scenario for his hospital stay. Following are several procedures performed on him in an attempt to acquire a definitive diagnosis: (1) flexible esophagoscopy with ultrasound examination; (2) flexible colonoscopy, proximal to splenic flexure, with removal of two polyps; and (3) liver biopsy. From blood tests performed by the ED physician, it was determined that Mr. Metcalf was severely anemic. As a result, he was given a blood transfusion. Using the most recent CPT-4 manual, code these four procedures.

4. The use of modifiers in CPT coding can indicate that a service or procedure has been altered by some specific circumstance, but without changing its definition or code. Let's assume that the liver biopsy took more time than is typically required. Identify which modifier would be used in this example.

5. On the last day of his hospitalization, Mr. Metcalf underwent a needle biopsy of the prostate. What would be the correct CPT code for this procedure?
   a. 55700
   b. 55705
   c. 55720
   d. 55725

6. _____ True or False: Wilson Metcalf was discharged from the hospital on day 4. The physician spent a total of 45 minutes documenting the medical record and then discussing test results, prognoses, and medication requirements with the patient and his son. The correct CPT code for hospital discharge would be 99238.

➤ • Close Mr. Metcalf's chart and **Return to Map**.

Exercise 3

CD-ROM Activity—CPT Coding Assignment 3

20 minutes

- From the patient list, choose **Teresa Hernandez**. (*Note:* If you have exited the program, sign back in and select Teresa Hernandez from the patient list.)

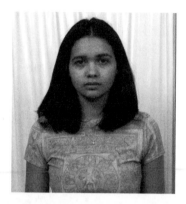

Teresa Hernandez

- Click on the **Billing and Coding** office.

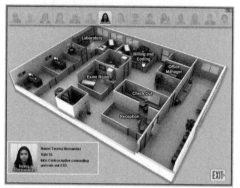

Click on Billing and Coding.

- Choose **Charts**, click on the **Patient Medical Information** tab, and select **1-Progress Notes**.

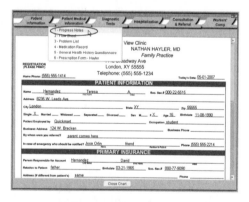

Click on 1-Progress Notes.

- Review the Progress Notes for 05-01-2007.
- Click **Close Chart** and select **Encounter Form** under the View heading.

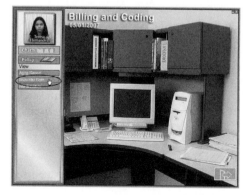

Click on Encounter Form.

1. List and code all procedures/services that were performed on this date.

2. Using your CPT manual, research the list of modifiers in Appendix A. Let's assume that Teresa is a Level V established patient. Because of her multiple concurrent problems, her visit (including examination, assessment, and counseling with the patient and her parents) took longer than usual—90 minutes. Is a modifier applicable to this situation? If so, what modifier should be used?

3. Teresa will return in 3 weeks for a Pap test. What CPT code should be used for this test?

4. _____ True or False: Teresa was given a prescription for a "seasonal oral contraceptive pack." This does not require a CPT code.

Diagnostic Coding

Reading Assignment: Chapter 45—Medical Coding
  • Diagnostic Coding

Patients: Jose Imero, Kevin McKinzie

Objectives:

- Describe the format and use of International Classification of Diseases, Ninth Revision, Clinical Modification (ICD-9-CM) codes.
- Demonstrate how fourth and fifth digits are used with ICD-9-CM codes.
- Demonstrate how to locate an accurate ICD-9-CM code.
- Demonstrate an understanding of the ICD-9-CM coding process by accurately coding patients' diagnoses to the greatest degree of specificity.

Exercise 1

Writing Activity—Applying Accurate Codes to the Diagnoses Listed on the Encounter Form

10 minutes

1. Using the most recent edition of the ICD-9-CM codebook and the coding steps presented in the textbook, insert the correct diagnosis codes for each of the given conditions listed on the form below. If there is not enough information to code to the highest degree of specificity to assign a fourth and/or fifth digit, insert an X in place of the fourth and/or fifth digits. (*Example:* If the diagnosis is "malnutrition," and no additional information is available for coding more specifically, list the code as 263.XX.)

___ Abscess	___ Asthma	___ Depression	___ Hematuria	___ Pregnancy
___ Abrasion-Sup.Injury	___ Backache	___ Dermatitis	___ Hemorrhoids	___ Rectal Bleed
___ Acne	___ Breast Mass	___ Diabetes*	___ HIV	___ Sinusitis
___ Alcohol Abuse	___ Bronchitis	___ Diarrhea	___ Hypertension	___ STD _____
___ Allergic Reaction	___ Bursitis	___ Dysmenorrheal	___ Hypothyroidism	___ Tendonitis
___ Amenorrhea	___ CAD	___ Ear Impaction	___ IBS	___ UTI
___ Anemia	___ Chest Pain	___ Fatigue	___ Low Back Pain	___ URI
___ Anxiety	___ CHF	___ Fever	___ Lymphadenopathy	___ Vaginitis
___ Annual GYN exam	___ Conjunctivitis	___ Fracture	___ Nausea/Vomiting	___ Well Baby/Child
___ Annual PE	___ COPD	___ Gastritis	___ Obesity	___ Weight Loss
___ Arrhythmia	___ Contraception	___ Gastroenteritis	___ Osteoporosis	___ Otitis Media
___ Arthritis	___ Cough	___ Gout	___ Pharyngitis	___ Elevated BP
___ ASHD	___ CVA	___ Headache	___ Pneumonia	___
				___

Exercise 2

Writing Activity—Diagnostic Coding for Jose Imero

🕐 15 minutes

- Sign in to Mountain View Clinic.
- Select **Jose Imero** from the patient list.

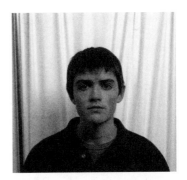

Jose Imero

- Enter the **Exam Room** from the office map.

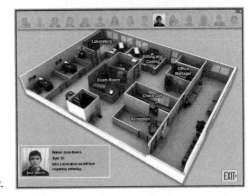

Click on Exam Room.

- In the Exam Room, select **Exam Notes** (under View).

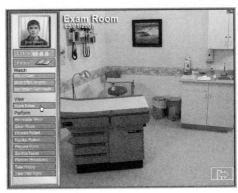

Click on Exam Notes.

1. Based on the Exam Notes, what is (are) the diagnosis(es) for this patient?

2. The first step in coding this diagnosis is to identify the _____ and

locate it in the _____.

3. The main term of this patient's diagnosis is:
   a. laceration.
   b. left foot.
   c. plantar surface.
   d. inner aspect.

4. When you located the main term in the ICD-9-CM, what did you learn?

5. After completing the step in question 4, what code(s) did you locate?

6. After cross-referencing the code(s) to the tabular section and coding the diagnosis to the greatest degree of specificity, what is the correct primary code that should be reported in block 21 of the CMS-1500 claim?

7. What is the rule for using E codes on an insurance claim?

➤ • Close the Exam Notes, click on the exit arrow, and select **Return to Map**.

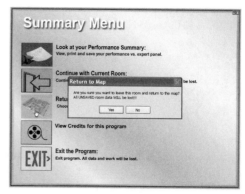

Return to Map

Exercise 3

 CD-ROM Activity—Diagnostic Coding for Kevin McKinzie

 20 minutes

- Choose **Kevin McKinzie** from the patient list. (*Note:* If you have exited the program, sign back in to Mountain View Clinic and choose Kevin McKinzie from the patient list.)

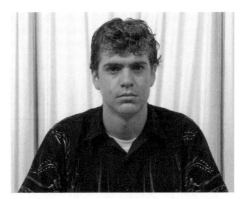

Kevin McKinzie

- On the office map, highlight and click on **Exam Room**.

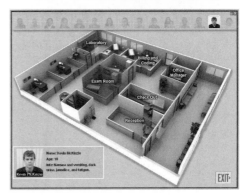

Click on Exam Room.

- In the Exam Room, select **Patient Interview** (under View).

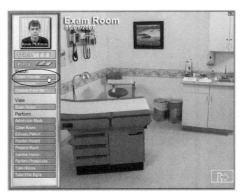

Click on Patient Interview.

- At the end of the video, click **Close** to return to the Exam Room.
- Now select and review this patient's Exam Notes.

1. During the patient interview, what symptoms does the patient claim to have?

2. In the Exam Notes for this patient, what health problems does the physician document under "Impression"?

3. One entry in the Exam Notes under "Impression" is worded as as "R/O hepatitis, mono." What is the rule about coding an entry like this?

4. When should an ICD-9 code be assigned to impressions documented as symptoms or worded as "rule out"?

➤ • Click **Finish** to close the Exam Notes. Click on the exit arrow and select **Return to Map**.
 • Continuing with patient Kevin McKinzie, click on **Billing and Coding** on the office map.
 • Click on **Encounter Form** and examine the diagnoses indicated for this patient.

5. True or False:

 a. _____ The diagnoses indicated on Kevin McKinzie's Encounter Form are the same as those documented under "Impression" in the Exam Notes.

 b. _____ The biller/coder should report the conditions/diagnoses documented in the patient's medical chart in block 21 of the CMS-1500 as opposed to those noted on the Encounter Form.

6. When the diagnoses listed on the Encounter Form are different from those documented in the medical record, the biller/coder should:
 a. report only the diagnosis codes noted on the Encounter Form.
 b. report only the diagnosis codes documented in the medical record.
 c. report both the diagnosis codes documented in the record and on the Encounter Form.
 d. report the discrepancy to the physician and ask for clarification regarding what specific diagnoses to code and report.
 e. insert an "addendum" to the medical record, adding the missing diagnoses codes from the Encounter Form.

7. Match each symptom or diagnosis with its correct ICD-9 code.

Symptom or Diagnosis	**ICD-9 Code**
_____ Dark urine	a. 780.79
_____ Nausea/vomiting	b. 787.01
_____ Fatigue	c. 788.9
_____ Asthma	d. 493.90
_____ Jaundice	e. 783.21
_____ Weight loss	f. 782.4

8. Note that "stomach pain" is not included in the "Symptom or Diagnosis" list in question 7. Why not?

9. Note that the physician did document "GI symptoms" under "Impression" in the Exam Notes. Can this condition be coded? Why or why not?

Medical Insurance

_____

⬯⬯ Reading Assignment: Chapter 46—Medical Insurance

Patients: Shaunti Begay, Louise Parlet, John R. Simmons, Janet Jones

Objectives:

- Apply managed care policies and procedures to office billing and coding.
- Use third-party guidelines for preparing insurance claims and collecting co-payments.
- Perform procedural coding.
- Perform diagnostic coding.
- Prepare a clean insurance claim form.

Exercise 1

 CD-ROM Activity—Verifying Insurance for a New Patient

 30 minutes

- Sign in to Mountain View Clinic.
- From the patient list, select **Shaunti Begay**.

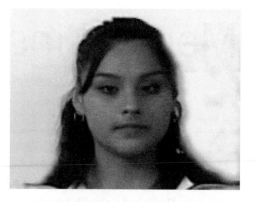

Shaunti Begay

- On the office map, highlight and click on **Reception**.

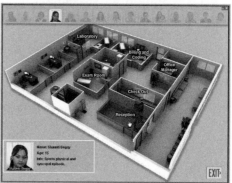

Click on Reception.

- At the Reception desk, click on **Policy** to open the office Policy Manual.

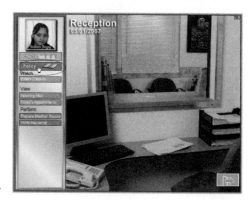

Click on Policy.

- Type "17" in the search bar and click the magnifying glass. This will take you to page 17 of the Policy Manual. Scroll up to adjust the page and read the policies that apply when patients have insurance coverage that is not accepted by the medical practice.

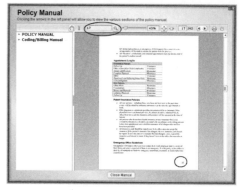

Search for page 17.

1. According to the Policy Manual, what information should be obtained from the patient when the appointment is made?

2. Why is it important for the medical assistant to verify *at the time the appointment is made* whether the office is a preferred provider with the patient's insurance?

➡ • Scroll up to page 14 of the Policy Manual and read the section on Telephone Policies.

3. What does the Policy Manual state about collecting payments, co-pays, and percentages of charges for patient visits?

➡ • Click **Close Manual** to return to the Reception desk.
  • Click on **Patient Check-In** to view the video of Shaunti's arrival at the clinic.

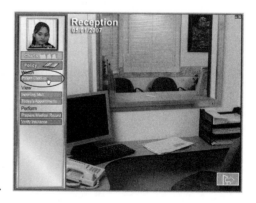

Click on Patient Check-In.

  • At the end of the video, click **Close** to return to the Reception desk.

→ • At the Reception desk, click on **Verify Insurance** to obtain the required information for Shaunti's visit.

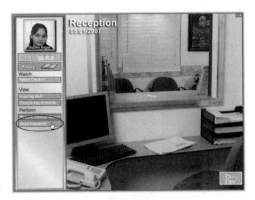

Click on Verify Insurance.

• Select the appropriate question to ask Shaunti regarding her insurance; then review the Insurance Cards on the next screen.

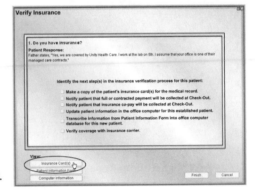

Review the Insurance Cards.

• Click **Finish** to return to the Reception desk.
• Click again on **Policy** to reopen the Policy Manual.
• From the menu on the left side of the screen, click on the arrow next to **Coding/Billing Manual** to view the additional headings for that section of the Policy Manual.
• Click the arrow next to **Financial Policy** and select **Accepted Insurance Carriers** from the list.

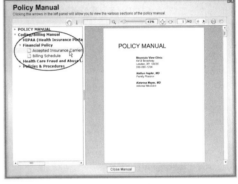

Click Accepted Insurance Carriers.

• Click **Close Manual** to return to the Reception desk.

4. Was Kristin correct in stating that Mountain View Clinic was not a participating provider for Shaunti's insurance plan?

5. What did Shaunti's mother say about the information she gave the receptionist regarding their insurance coverage when she made the appointment?

6. What steps should the medical assistant have taken to avoid the confusion that occurred when Shaunti checked in?

- Click the exit arrow to leave the Reception desk.
- From the Summary Menu, select **Return to Map**.

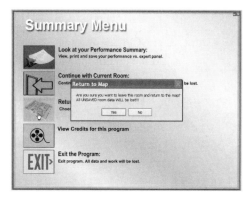

Click Return to Map.

Exercise 2

 CD-ROM Activity—Obtaining a Referral for an Established Patient

 30 minutes

- Select **Louise Parlet** from the patient list. (*Note:* If you have exited the program, sign in again to Mountain View Clinic and select Louise Parlet from the patient list.)

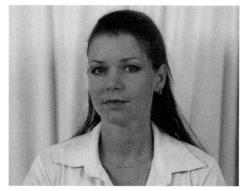

Louise Parlet

- On the office map, highlight and click on **Check Out**.

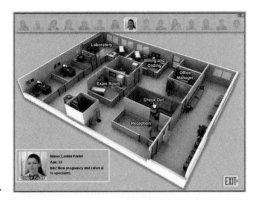

Click on Check Out.

- At the desk, click on **Patient Check-Out** to view the video.

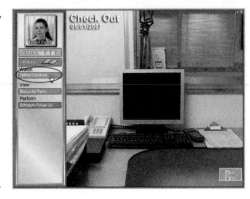

Click on Patient Check-Out.

- At the end of the video, click **Close** to return to the desk.

1. Why is it important that the medical assistant help Ms. Parlet obtain approval from her insurance company for the referral to Dr. Lockett?

2. After receiving the precertification verification number, how should the medical assistant handle the verification number?

- Next, click on **Charts** to open Ms. Parlet's medical record.
- Under the **Patient Medical Information** tab, select **3-Progress Notes** and read Dr. Hayler's notes regarding the examination.

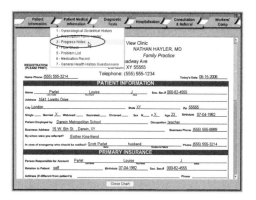

Click on 3-Progress Notes.

3. What instructions does Dr. Hayler give about the results of the lab work? How do these instructions affect the insurance coverage?

- Click **Close Chart** to return to the Check Out desk.
- Click the exit arrow; from the Summary Menu, select **Return to Map**.

Exercise 3

  CD-ROM Activity—Coding an Office Visit of a New Adult Patient

30 minutes

- Select **John R. Simmons** from the patient list. (*Note:* If you have exited the program, sign in again to Mountain View Clinic and select John R. Simmons from the patient list.)

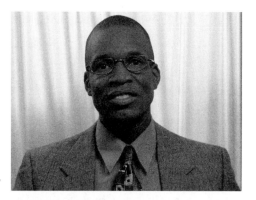

John R. Simmons

- On the office map, highlight and click on **Billing and Coding**.

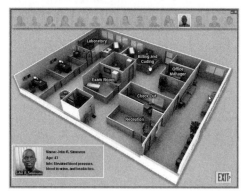

Click on Billing and Coding.

→ • At the Billing and Coding desk, click on **Encounter Form** to view the diagnostic and procedural information for Dr. Simmons' visit.

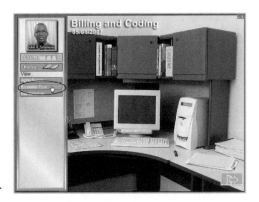

Click on Encounter Form.

1. In the ICD-9 section of the Encounter Form, which diagnoses are checked off for Dr. Simmons' visit?

2. Which of these diagnoses should receive an ICD-9 code? If there are any diagnoses that should not be coded, explain why not.

3. When should the home-obtained hemoccult testing be billed and coded? Explain your answer.

→ • Click **Finish** to close the Encounter Form and return to the Billing and Coding desk.

• Click on **Charts** to open Dr. Simmons' medical record and select **5-Insurance Cards** from under the **Patient Information** tab.

4. Using the information on the insurance cards found in the medical record, what is the co-pay on the patient's insurance? What is the payment rate on the secondary insurance?

5. What is meant by PCP?

6. What is meant by POS?

- Click **Close Chart** to return to the Billing and Coding desk.
- Click the exit arrow; from the Summary Menu, select **Return to Map**.

Exercise 4

 CD-ROM Activity—Insurance Versus Workers' Compensation Claims

 15 minutes

- From the patient list, select **Janet Jones**. (*Note:* If you have exited the program, sign in again to Mountain View Clinic and select Janet Jones from the patient list.)

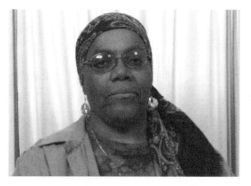

Janet Jones

- On the office map, highlight and click on **Billing and Coding**.

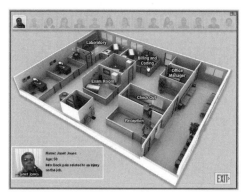

Click on Billing and Coding.

- Click on **Charts** to open Janet Jones' medical record.
- Next, click on the **Patient Information** tab.

1. You will notice that in Ms. Jones' medical record, there is no information about private insurance coverage. Why is this important for this case?

2. What information is needed for a Workers' Compensation claim that is not needed for a private insurance claim?

→ • Now click on the tab labeled **Workers' Comp**.

3. What information do you find under this tab in Ms. Jones' medical record?

4. If the Workers' Compensation carrier declares Ms. Jones' claim to be nonindustrial and refuses to pay it, is Mountain View Clinic required to write off the balance?